THE UNBOTHERED BUTTON

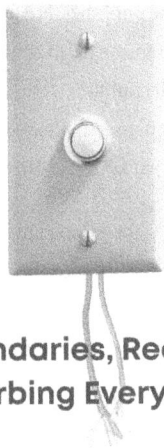

How to Set Boundaries, Reclaim Your Peace, and Stop Absorbing Everyone Else's Chaos

Dr. Shiloh Werkmeister

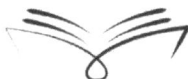

LITTLE BLACK BOOK

PUBLISHING

St Louis, MO

Cover photo by Morgan Ramsour

Published by LBB Publishing. An imprint of Little Black Book: Women in Business

Ebook ISBN: 978-1-962417-28-0

Paperback ISBN: 978-1-962417-29-7

Hardcover ISBN: 978-1-962417-30-3

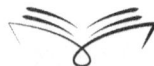

LITTLE BLACK BOOK
PUBLISHING

ALSO BY

Dr. Shiloh Werkmeister

Conversational Boundaries

Emotion Explorers

Go Crazy Inside the Lines

PRAISE FOR

The Unbothered Button

As a Christian leader, busy professional, and natural empath, I have searched in every decade of my life for the line between loving others like Jesus and giving all I have to the point of burnout.

A number of years ago, I hit my breaking point. With a frazzled nervous system and broken heart, I set out on a quest to learn HOW to live the abundant life Jesus has for me in my daily life. Through the Bible, counseling, and a myriad of books, I sought to find and to protect my peace. I am still on that journey daily.

When I met Dr. Werkmeister, I immediately recognized her unique, God-given gift to combine both spiritual wisdom from the Word of God with medical expertise to help people like me — those searching for healthy nervous systems, leading to the boldness and confidence needed to live out the calling God has placed on their lives.

Now she brings this wisdom to so many through her winsome book, The Unbothered Button. If you are like me, looking for practical tips and inspiration for real-life change to enjoy unshakable peace, this is the book for you! Dr. Werkmeister powerfully shares how to reclaim your energy, your time, and your peace in order to honor the calling on your life — all while loving yourself AND others. I cannot recommend it more highly!

—Sarah Guldalian, Award-Winning Producer, Writer, Speaker, & Ministry Leader, Top Notch Brand Co.

The Unbothered Button is more than a book—it's a breath of fresh air for anyone who's ever felt emotionally hijacked by other people's drama. Dr. Shiloh Werkmeister offers a powerful, compassionate reminder that you don't have to answer every knock on your emotional door.

What I loved most is that it's not about shutting down or building walls—it's about learning how to set healthy, sacred boundaries that protect your peace without compromising your heart. The idea of "disconnecting your emotional doorbell" hit me right in the gut (in the best way). It gave language to something I've been trying to do for years—but didn't know how.

Dr. Shiloh blends science, soul, and real-life wisdom in a way that feels both practical and deeply validating. I saw myself in the examples, and for once, I didn't feel broken—I felt understood.

This is an important book for everyone, but as a Functional Health Practitioner working with women navigating midlife, I found it especially helpful. So many of my clients are dealing with burnout, over-giving, and nervous system overload—The Unbothered Button offers exactly the kind of support and language they need to begin reclaiming their peace and power.

If you're ready to stop letting chaos, guilt, or manipulation run your life, this book shows you how to step into your strength without losing your softness.

– Laini Gray, FDNP, Gray Star Health & Fitness

Just when I thought I had my boundaries figured out, this book cracked me wide open. It's powerful, perspective-shifting, and deeply reflective. It made me feel, think, and realize there's still more work to do—and that's a gift. This isn't just a book you read; it's a book you work through. One that has the potential to transform you, if you let it.

–April B., Becoming Unbothered Participant

I'm looking forward to implementing the pause protocol into my life. I feel like it is something that could drastically reframe my mindset and my life.

–Danielle L., Becoming Unbothered Participant

I wish I would have had the tools mentioned in the book earlier in my life. The book is written with encouragement, reminding us that rewiring our thinking takes time and compassion. The examples and stories in the book make it "real". The chapters are filled with a lot of information, but the "Try this Toolkit" component allows time to pause and reflect. I see this as a book worth reading and rereading throughout life.

One of my many favorite statements in the book, "Becoming unbothered is learning to reframe your internal narrative. You don't have to silence your thoughts. You just have to start questioning them."

–Charlotte Gray, Educator

AUDIOBOOK BONUS

Listen While You Heal

Get the Free Audiobook, Delivered through an Exclusive Private Podcast!

If you're the kind of person who learns best by listening, I've got you.

You can now access a **private podcast version** of *The Unbothered Button*, narrated by me (Dr. Shiloh)–with extra commentary, behind-the-scenes insights, and calming narration you can take on a walk, to the gym, or into your nighttime wind-down.

- Easy access on your favorite podcast app

- Author-narrated, personal and heartfelt (Sass included!)

- Exclusive bonus reflections not found in the book

Free with email sign-up here:

CONTENTS

For every soul who has quietly carried the weight of others' expectations, may you finally put it down and walk unbothered. Your courage changes everything.

And for Mikayla–watching you grow into your power has been one of my life's greatest privileges. May you always protect your peace, trust your instincts, and never let the world convince you to shrink. This book is a blueprint for the fire I already see in you.

You are not required to set yourself on fire to keep others warm.

— Unknown

CHAPTER 1
YOUR BUTTONS AREN'T THE PROBLEM

L et me tell you a quick story. It's a simple story about a doorbell, but, for me, it was the catalyst for a whole new way of thinking. I hope this story, and the resulting mindset shift, will have a profound effect on you too.

Recently, I have been staying at my grandmother's house while my home was being renovated. Her name is Virginia, but everyone who loves her calls her GG. Now, GG's house isn't one of those tiny little grandma cottages with lace curtains and fresh apple pie on the windowsill. No, ma'am. Her house is a place full of quirks and mysteries.

GG's house is *big*. Like, walkie-talkie big. Like, you-could-yell-and-still-not-be-heard big. In fact, she even had one of those built-in intercom systems from the '80s wired into the walls, each room with a little speaker and button, like we were living in a sitcom. It hasn't worked in years, but it's still there. A relic from a time when the house needed help *communicating with itself*.

And honestly? That's a whole sermon right there.

GG's house also didn't smell like cookies or fresh-baked pies or anything you'd find in a Hallmark movie. Nope. Her house smelled like onions. Always onions. She was—how do I say this gently?—a *disaster* in the kitchen. I am fairly certain she knew cooking wasn't her forte and chose not to be bothered by this. If you ever saw her cooking, you'd feel compelled to call in backup. I remember one time in particular when GG decided to make soup, which, as it turns out, was her code word for dumping all the leftovers in her refrigerator into a pot, adding ketchup, some water, and voilà. Even the dog refused to eat it.

But if you sat with her while she stirred a pot of something *questionable*, you'd be fed in all the ways that mattered. She was present. She was warm. She made you feel like your feelings had a place to sit down and stay for a while. She loved Jesus. And cared not just for her family but her community and neighbors. She was full of homespun wisdom and a dry sense of humor. Sometimes the best teachers don't even realize they are teaching.

Growing up, her house, onion-scented and oversized, was a place where the chaos of the world softened. Not because it was peaceful in the Pinterest sense, but because GG was the kind of person who made *you* feel peaceful. At the time of this writing, GG is still alive and kicking, ninety-six years young, and full of feisty wit. She probably doesn't realize it, but I have learned a lot by watching how she navigates the world.

One afternoon, I was all the way in the back of the house, probably reading, sipping tea, and living my best introverted life, when someone came to the front door. Apparently, they knocked. They rang the doorbell. Then they rang it again. And again. And according to a neighbor, they started getting heated, full-on angry knocking, pacing on the porch like they were rehearsing a monologue, probably convinced I was ignoring them on purpose.

But here's the kicker. The doorbell didn't work. It had been disconnected years ago. So, no matter how many times they pushed that little button, no chime, no ding-dong, no signal. Imagine what that must have felt like for the button pusher. Incredibly frustrating. But for me, it had the opposite effect. I stayed calm. I stayed quiet. I stayed *unbothered* in the back bedroom.

When I finally found out someone had been furiously banging and button-mashing on GG's front porch, I didn't feel bad. I wasn't being rude. I genuinely didn't hear them. Because no matter how desperately they wanted a response from me, **the signal didn't reach me.**

That's when it hit me. **This is the emotional boundary I want in my life.** Right here.

How many times in our lives do people come up to our emotional front porch with all the energy of a frustrated Amazon driver, demanding we answer their urgency? They push the guilt button. They knock with passive aggression. They ring the doorbell of old childhood wounds. You know, the ones labeled, *you're too much, you're selfish, you owe me.*

And if your emotional doorbell is still connected, guess what? You hear every single ring. You *feel* every single knock. You drop what you're doing. You scramble to answer. You spiral.

But here's the truth. **You are allowed to disconnect that doorbell.** If you're exhausted from being everyone's emotional punching bag... If you always leave conversations replaying what you *should* have said... If your nervous system is in a constant state of defense... This book will change your life by teaching you how to disconnect your buttons, just like GG's doorbell. I call it the Unbothered Button, an invisible boundary between peace and chaos.

If you've ever felt emotionally hijacked, stuck in over-thinking, triggered by people who *shouldn't matter,* or exhausted by your own reactions, you're in the right place. You don't need to shut down to survive. You need to rewire your system.

Throughout this book, I'll walk you through the framework I developed to help clients (and myself) disconnect emotional buttons, reclaim peace, and stay grounded no matter who's pushing. And you'll learn how to be powerful in the most unshakable way; with calm, clear, unapologetic energy. You've spent enough of your life reacting. Now it's time to rewire. Let's begin.

Signs your emotional doorbell is still connected

Let's do a quick gut check. These are some common signs that someone, or multiple someones, still have emotional access to you, whether you've realized it or not. This isn't an exhaustive list, and you don't need to check every box to know it's time to make a change. This is just a starting point. A mirror, not a judgment.

If you find yourself nodding along to even *one or two* of these, take a deep breath. You're not broken. You're just wired for responsiveness in a world that *rewards over-functioning and punishes rest*. But you can rewire that. You *will*. The following list can help you recognize whether or not you may need to disconnect yourself from the buttons that keep triggering you. Mark any that sound familiar.

☐ You say *yes* to things you *resent* five minutes later.

☐ You feel physically uneasy when someone sends a vague, *Can we talk?* text.

☐ You've ever rehearsed your boundaries in your head like it's a courtroom testimony.

☐ You replay conversations days (or *weeks*) later, trying to decode whether you were too much, not enough, or just completely misunderstood.

☐ You abandon your plans to tend to someone else's chaos, even though they never return the favor.

☐ You feel emotionally exhausted after short interactions that *should've* been neutral.

☐ You second-guess your intuition and defer to other people's comfort over your own clarity.

Did you have a few checkmarks? Maybe more than a few? Maybe a lot?

You're not alone. Many of us were raised to be polite instead of powerful. To be pleasant instead of being present with our own needs. But when your peace is constantly up for grabs, you stop feeling like *yourself* and start feeling like a 24/7 crisis manager for other people's emotions. That stops here.

What does that actually mean?

Disconnecting the emotional doorbell doesn't mean you become cold. It doesn't mean you stop caring. In fact, people who master this skill are often deeply feeling, empathetic, and intuitive. It's precisely because they feel so much that they *have* to learn how not to absorb every toxic drop of the world around them. Becoming unbothered means *you stop being available to chaos*. It means you create a little sacred space between someone else's *button-pushing behavior* and your *automatic reaction*. It's a radical act of self-protection. It says, *I can still care deeply, without letting your chaos live inside me.*

Let's be honest, we all have buttons. For some of us, it's when someone questions our worth. For others, it's being ignored, dismissed, or made to feel like we're *too sensitive*. And if you're anything like me, your buttons didn't appear overnight. They were installed over years of conditioning, trauma, people-pleasing, and situations where it was safer to be small and compliant than real and unapologetic. But you know what? Those buttons aren't permanent fixtures.

They're wires you can trace, name, and gently start to pull out. You can do the emotional equivalent of walking up to your own wiring system and saying, *Yeah, we're not using this anymore.*

Emotional boundaries are not walls.

They're filters. They're intelligent, soul-saving systems that ask, *Is this mine to carry? Does this align with my peace? Am I responding... or just reacting?*

When you start to get real about your emotional boundaries, you stop answering to every knock. You stop letting people shake your foundation every time they have a bad day. You stop being the emotional 9-1-1 dispatcher for people who refuse to take accountability.

Emotional sovereignty is a skill.

It takes work to stop reacting out of habit. It takes courage to let people be uncomfortable with your boundaries. It takes *practice* to sit in the stillness of not responding.

Because here's what no one tells you. **Constant button pushing doesn't just mess with your head–it fries your nervous system.** When someone guilt-trips you, love-bombs you, shames you, or flips from kind to cruel in a heartbeat, your body feels it before your brain does.

Your heart rate spikes. Your muscles tense. Your chest tightens, as if bracing for an emotional impact. You go from peaceful to panicked in a single sentence. And your nervous system, bless it, can't tell if you're in a heated conversation or being chased by a bear.

It doesn't care that it's *just a text* or *just your mom* or *just your ex.* It reacts like something is threatening your safety, because emotionally, it is.

This is why boundaries aren't just emotional. They're physiological. You're not overreacting. You're overstimulated. And that's not weakness. That's wisdom waiting to be honored.

What's happening in your body when your buttons get pushed?

You might think someone *just made a comment,* but your body experienced it as a threat. When emotional buttons get pushed, especially the ones tied to old trauma, people-pleasing, or deep insecurities, your nervous system lights up like it's DEFCON 1.

Here's what's actually going on inside you. Let's start with your brain. The amygdala (your fear detector) goes, *Oh no, we've been here before.* It sends out a panic signal before your rational brain even has a chance to weigh in. The prefrontal cortex (your logical, calm decision-maker) gets *hijacked*, which is why you can't think straight or form a decent comeback until hours later in the shower.

Meanwhile, in your body, there's a whole other process happening. Your heart rate increases. Your body thinks you need to run or fight. Breathing becomes shallow, and with less oxygen reaching your brain, it leads to foggy thinking. Your muscles tense up. Hello, jaw clenching, shoulder knots, and tension headaches. And your digestive system slows, which is why stress can make you nauseous, bloated, or irregular.

The fallout from this stress on your nervous system is intense. If you're constantly in this reactive state, your body gets stuck in survival mode. That's where burnout, chronic fatigue, migraines, anxiety, and even autoimmune flares can sneak in. It's not *just stress*. It's a *dysregulated nervous system trying to protect you from emotional chaos.*

The good news is there's a solution. Boundaries. Clarity. Emotional disconnection from people who think they own access to you. It's not just mental health. It's whole body health.

Over time, you realize that just because someone pushes doesn't mean you have to move. Just because they're loud doesn't mean they're right. Just because they're disappointed doesn't mean you're wrong.

And that, my friend, is what it means to be **unbothered**. It's not about building walls. It's about building *wisdom*. It's about knowing who gets access to your energy, your peace, your nervous system. And it's about being so grounded in your truth that you don't need to run to the door every time someone shows up uninvited, asking you to abandon yourself.

So from here on out, I want you to think of every button someone tries to push as a disconnected doorbell. They might press it. They might press it *hard*. They might stand there frustrated that you're not reacting like you used to.

But you? You're in the back of the house. Sipping your tea. Listening to your intuition. Living your life. **Unbothered.**

In this book, we're going to disconnect some serious doorbells. You'll learn how to stop being available to nonsense, how to become emotionally *unbothered* (not cold, let's be clear, we still love deeply over here), and how to protect your peace like it's your job. Because it kinda is.

In the chapters ahead, we're going to trace the wires, identify the voices that programmed your buttons, and slowly start unplugging from what no longer serves you. You'll learn how to hold boundaries without spiraling. How to stay soft *and* strong. And how to become unshakably rooted in your peace.

I promise to keep it honest, a little spicy, and packed with tools that actually work. No fluff. No filler. Just clarity, boundaries, and a few mic drops.

Ready to uninstall some buttons? Let's go.

Try This: Button Mapping

Before we wrap up this chapter, I want you to do something brave.

Take a few minutes, just you and a notebook, or even the notes app on your phone, and try this quick reflection. You don't have to get it perfect. You don't have to have all the answers. Just start where you are. Because awareness... that's the beginning of freedom.

We're going to map out the emotional buttons that are still connected. Take three minutes and work through the following steps.

Step 1: Who pushes your buttons the most?
Write down a few names. Be honest. This could be a partner, parent, friend, boss, sibling, or even that one client who *always* seems to think they're the exception to your boundaries. Don't overthink it. Go with your gut.

Step 2: What *exactly* are they pressing?
Ask yourself: *What stories or phrases do they use that make you feel small, guilty, or reactive?* Do they question your character, your priorities, or your worth in subtle (or not-so-subtle) ways? What emotional tone tends to get under your skin? Does it sound like disappointment, blame, silence, or neediness? And perhaps most importantly, are they activating an old role you used to play without even realizing it? Maybe the *good girl, the fixer, the*

peacekeeper, or *the one who always keeps the peace no matter the cost.*

Step 3: What is your automatic response?
Notice how your body and behavior react when your button is pushed. Do you fawn? Apologize? Over-explain? Numb out? Do you shrink, rage, cry, freeze, or try to fix?

Be gentle with yourself here. These responses aren't character flaws. They're survival strategies that worked once. You're not weak. You're just tired of being on high alert.

Step 4: Ask the big question. What would happen if this button didn't work anymore?
Visualize that doorbell being unplugged. The person still pushes it, but you don't answer. You don't even *hear* it. How would your day feel? Your week? Your life? What version of you would show up if you weren't constantly being pulled out of alignment?

This is your first act of becoming unbothered. Not disconnected from life, but deeply connected to *yourself*. You've spent enough time emotionally on-call. You've earned the right to let the doorbell ring...and keep sipping your tea.

Why We Need the Unbothered Button

You might be wondering, *Okay, but is this really that big of a deal? Does it actually matter if I keep reacting to people emotionally?*

Yes. It matters more than most people realize.

The constant emotional overstimulation from others, being pulled into guilt, drama, manipulation, or chronic people-pleasing, isn't just annoying. It's *destructive*. Chronic emotional stress has been linked to anxiety, depression, sleep disorders, hormonal imbalances, and even autoimmune issues. Emotional reactivity keeps your brain in survival mode, your body in tension, and your spirit in a permanent state of alert.

Let me say it plainly. **Living in a constant state of emotional defense wears you out.**

It's not just your mood that suffers. It's your ability to focus. To be present with your kids. To enjoy your work. To have a conversation without bracing for conflict. To feel peace in your own skin.

We don't always recognize this for what it is, because most of us have *normalized the dysfunction*. We've been taught that self-abandonment is the price of being *kind*. That burnout is just part of being a good mom, a loyal partner, a hard worker.

But no more. This book is here to give you a way out. Not just another list of *boundary tips*, but a full-on rewiring.

Anchoring Truth

When appropriate, I will be dropping a little bit of spiritual truth on you throughout this book. These verses are here to remind you that protecting your peace isn't just a mindset shift. It's a spiritual act.

Above all else, guard your heart, for everything you do flows from it. – Proverbs 4:23

Your worth was never meant to be negotiated, and your boundaries aren't just mental tools. They are sacred guardrails that honor the calling on your life. **The Unbothered Button is more than a metaphor.** It's a step-by-step system to help you disconnect the emotional triggers that have run your life for far too long.

This book will teach you how to spot the buttons and who installed them. Regulate your nervous system in real-time. Create boundaries that don't buckle under pressure. Best of all, you will learn how to reclaim your energy, your time, and your peace.

In the chapters that follow, you'll learn how to identify the emotional buttons that keep getting pushed, understand why they exist, and begin the process of disconnecting them for good. We'll dive into the psychology behind emotional reactions, explore the patterns that keep you stuck, and walk through my B.U.T.T.O.N. Framework™, designed to help you build internal strength, set powerful boundaries, and reclaim your peace. Each chapter offers practical tools, real-life insights, and reflection prompts to guide your transformation. By the end of this book, you'll not only understand how to stop giving others access to your emotional control panel. You'll feel grounded in your ability to live unbothered, no matter what chaos surrounds you. When I say unbothered, I don't mean checked out or cold or distant. I mean grounded. I mean calm, even when things get loud. I mean fully present without letting other people pull your strings.

And you'll do it with heart. With humor. With your humanity fully intact. No harsh walls. No emotional shutdown. Just clarity, alignment, and calm confidence. You don't have to keep living on edge. There's another way. And it starts here. It's time to stop giving out access to your nervous system like it's free Wi-Fi. Let's get to work. This first step isn't about becoming someone new. It's about finally becoming someone true—to yourself.

PART I

Understanding Your Buttons

Until you make the unconscious conscious, it will direct your life and you will call it fate.

— Carl Jung

CHAPTER 2
EMOTIONAL BUTTONS: WHAT ARE THEY?

I magine getting cut off in traffic, and before you even think, your heart is racing, your hand's on the horn, and you're yelling into the air. That's not you. It's your wiring reacting faster than your wisdom. By now, you're probably starting to realize... you've got buttons.

Not literal ones–though if emotional boundaries could be installed like smart home tech, I'd be first in line. I'm talking about the invisible, internal buttons people seem to find with uncanny precision. And when they do? Boom–your nervous system, mood, and sense of peace all detonate at once.

So what *are* emotional buttons, really?

Let's start with something you already know. People can get under your skin. Some do it intentionally. Others do it just by being themselves. Either way, you end up spiraling–angry, anxious, defensive, ashamed. You might obsess over the conversation later, unable to shake what was said or how you felt.

These are emotional buttons. They're the psychological triggers wired into you over time, built from a mix of childhood conditioning, trauma, social expectations, and repeated patterns in relationships. They're not defects. They're signals. They show up when something in your nervous system says, *Hey, this isn't safe.* Even if it's just a look. A comment. A text that says, *Can we talk?*

An *emotional button* is a vulnerable spot wired to your nervous system. When someone pushes it, on purpose or not, it activates an automatic response. Cue people-pleasing, defensiveness, over-explaining, withdrawal, guilt, or even rage. The more history behind the button, the more reactive the response.

You might think your buttons are flaws. That if you could just *be less sensitive*, you wouldn't get so rattled. But the truth is, emotional buttons are shaped by experience, especially early ones. They're survival strategies that your body learned to keep you safe.

Think about it. If you grew up in a home where expressing anger meant being punished or ignored, your body learned that suppressing your needs was safer. So when someone today raises their voice, your nervous system doesn't just hear a disagreement. It hears danger. And that button gets pushed.

These buttons often form during childhood, but they can also show up after toxic relationships, traumatic events, or repeated invalidation. They become subconscious pathways that light up under stress.

When My *Too Much* Button Got Pushed

Let me tell you a story that still makes me shake my head and reminds me how deep these emotional buttons run.

A while back, someone I once considered a close friend said something that hit me square in the chest. It was one of those offhand, passive-aggressive remarks that people like to dress up as *just being honest.*

She looked at me and said, *You know, not everyone wants to be analyzed all the time.*

Now, on the surface, that might sound harmless. Maybe even funny, if you're feeling generous. But the way she said it? It wasn't a joke. It wasn't curious or kind. It was sharp, deliberate, and aimed to sting. She wasn't offering feedback. She was trying to make me question myself.

And for a second, it worked. I felt my gut clench. That familiar, old ache of *Did I do something wrong?* bubbled up. My brain scrambled to check the conversation for clues. I started doubting my tone, replaying what I had said, wondering if I came across as intense, pushy, or judgmental.

But here's the thing, I hadn't said anything remotely analytical. I wasn't dissecting her feelings. I wasn't digging into her childhood or interpreting her behavior. I was just being present. Calm. Observant. Grounded.

Her comment wasn't a reflection of what I was doing. It was a reflection of how she *felt being seen by someone like me.*

I wasn't analyzing her. She was projecting. Because something in my clarity made her uncomfortable with her own emotional messiness. My groundedness made her feel exposed, even though I hadn't lifted a finger.

And if you've ever had someone treat your calm presence like a threat, you know what I mean. That one sentence wasn't about me being *too much.* It was about her not being ready to be seen.

Still, it hit a button in me. The, *You're too intense. You make people uncomfortable. You always go too deep,* button. The one installed by years of being told that strength isn't feminine, that emotional honesty is impolite, and that wisdom is intimidating unless it comes with a soft voice and a side of self-deprecation.

In that moment, I had to pause and decide, was I going to shrink for her? Or was I going to stand in my truth? And that, right there, is the work. Not just noticing when your buttons are pushed, but learning how to stay rooted in yourself when they are.

Where Buttons Come From

So let's talk about how these buttons got installed in the first place. Because no one is born with a *too-much* button. Or a *fix-it-fast* button. Or a *don't-rock-the-boat* button.

These aren't flaws in your wiring. They're survival responses, shaped over time by experience, emotion, and repetition. For most of us, emotional buttons are installed early, before we even know what's happening. They come from the roles we had to play, the reactions we had to avoid, and the behaviors we learned that kept us safe, loved, or at least out of trouble.

If you grew up in a home where love had conditions, you might've developed a *people-pleasing* button. If anger was dangerous, you probably wired in a *keep the peace at all costs* button. If your emotions were dismissed or punished, you learned to stuff them down and smile, cue the *don't be dramatic* button.

These are not flaws. They are **evidence that your body tried to protect you**. But the problem is protection becomes overreaction when the system is stuck in old patterns. These buttons didn't start out as problems. They were solutions. They were your way of adapting to a world where you had to trade authenticity for acceptance. And when that happens long enough, your body begins to treat certain dynamics as threats, even when they're not. That's why a simple comment, a tone, or a pause in a text message can set off an entire cascade of panic or shutdown.

Repetition Becomes Programming

Think of it like this, your nervous system is a smart, sensitive computer. It stores data based on repeated exposure. If someone important to you repeatedly criticized you, dismissed you, or made you feel invisible, your system learned that similar behavior = danger.

And because the brain is wired for survival, not accuracy, it doesn't care if the current situation is totally different. It reacts *now* based on *then*. So you might be a grown, successful, emotionally aware woman, but if someone sighs or raises an eyebrow at the wrong time, your inner child might still panic and think, *I'm in trouble.*

This is how emotional buttons form. First, there's a repeated emotional pattern, something that happens often enough to leave an imprint. Maybe it's criticism, emotional withdrawal, or being made to feel responsible for someone else's mood. Then, your nervous system responds. It doesn't just store the memory; it stores the feeling. Your body starts to associate certain tones, words, or behaviors with danger, even if it's subtle. Over time, that pattern gets reinforced. Every similar experience confirms the reaction, and the button becomes more sensitive, more immediate. And before you know it, that button becomes hardwired, ready to fire instantly in adulthood, whether the threat is real or just *feels* familiar.

The Role of Conditioning

And then there's conditioning. Not from trauma necessarily, but from culture, religion, media, or gender roles.

Do any of these sound familiar? The belief that *good girls* don't set boundaries. The belief that mothers should be selfless and endlessly patient. How about the belief that it's better to stay quiet than make waves? Or that other people's comfort should always come before your truth.

These messages aren't just harmless suggestions. They're conditioning. Subtle, often unspoken rules we absorb over time. And the more we internalize them, the more likely we are to install emotional buttons that react any time we dare to defy them.

And so, *you adapted.* You made yourself smaller, softer, quieter, more agreeable. Until one day, you didn't even notice that your buttons weren't just being pushed... They were being *managed* by other people.

Awareness Example: Boys Don't Cry

Awareness is about naming the emotional wiring we inherited, often without consent. When Leo was seven, he scraped his knee at recess and burst into tears. His father knelt down, wiped the blood, and whispered harshly, *You're fine. Stop crying. Be a man.* That moment didn't just teach Leo to swallow his tears—it taught him that emotions were weakness. Now in his thirties, anytime his partner cries, Leo's chest tightens and he emotionally checks out. He doesn't mean to be cold, but his body interprets emotion as danger. The button was wired decades ago, and he never even realized it.

The Button → Trigger → Reaction Loop

Here's how it usually goes down.

Someone presses the button. They criticize you. Ignore you. Guilt-trip you. Roll their eyes. Demand access to what you didn't offer.

Your trigger fires. Your stomach drops. Your chest tightens. Your thoughts speed up. Your nervous system starts prepping for battle—or retreat.

You react. You fawn. You explain yourself. You get defensive. You shut down. You overfunction. You try to make it right—fast.

And just like that, you're no longer in your power. You're in your past.

This Isn't About Blame

Listen, having emotional buttons doesn't mean you're broken. It means you've been *human* in a world that hasn't always honored your humanity. We all have them. The question isn't whether you're triggered. The question is, **what do you do once you know that trigger is there?**

You can either keep reacting the same way and wondering why nothing changes...

Or you can start to recognize your buttons for what they are. Maps to healing. Signals from your body. Invitations to unplug what no longer serves you. When you start noticing your buttons without judgment, you create space to respond differently. Instead of jumping into your usual pattern of shutting down, snapping back, and over-apologizing, you can pause and ask: *What's really going on here?* That question changes everything.

The Big 5 Emotional Buttons

While everyone's emotional wiring is personal, there are a few buttons that show up *over and over again*, especially in women who've been conditioned to be everything for everyone.

Think of these as your emotional *hot keys*. When someone presses one, your system lights up like it's on fire, even if the moment feels small from the outside.

1. Rejection

This one sounds like: *You're not wanted.* It can be activated by silence, ghosting, being left out, or someone pulling away emotionally. Even a vague tone shift can set it off. If rejection is your button, you might scramble to reconnect, over-explain, or prove your worth before anyone even asks.

2. Criticism

This one whispers: *You can't get it wrong or you won't be loved.* It flares up when someone questions your choices, points out a flaw, or makes a *helpful suggestion* that wasn't asked for.

You might react with defensiveness, shame, or a perfectionism spiral that takes days to come down from.

3. Abandonment

This button is all about safety and stability. It says: *If I upset you, you'll leave, and I won't survive it.* It's especially common in people who had unpredictable caregivers or emotionally unavailable partners. This button often leads to fawning, people-pleasing, or tolerating bad behavior just to keep the peace.

4. Control

Ah, the illusion of safety. This one sounds like: *If I don't manage every detail, something bad will happen.* This button gets hit when plans change, people act unpredictably, or others don't respond the *right* way. You may feel anxious, irritable, or completely unmoored when this one's activated—and try to fix, plan, or overfunction your way back to calm.

5. Silencing

This one says: *Your voice doesn't matter. Don't speak, don't feel, don't need.* It shows up when someone talks over you, dismisses your feelings, or treats your emotions like a burden.

You might go quiet. Retreat. Shut down entirely—not because you don't have something to say, but because somewhere along the line, you learned it wasn't safe to say it.

If you saw yourself in one or all of these, take a breath. This doesn't mean you're weak or broken. It means your system is doing what it was trained to do. And now that you can name the buttons, you can *begin* to unhook them.

One of my clients once said, *It's like I get hijacked. I can feel myself reacting, but I can't stop it.* Yep. That's the nervous system firing off an old script. The goal of this book isn't to eliminate all your emotional responses. That's not realistic, or human. The goal is to help you *understand* them so you can unplug the ones that are causing unnecessary pain.

The Unbothered Button is not about becoming numb. It's about becoming so aware, so grounded, and so self-assured that your buttons stop working the way they used to. When that happens, you stop being baited by chaos. You stop apologizing for taking up space. You stop trying to fix everything. You start choosing *how* and *when* to engage. That's power.

Let's Normalize This

If any part of you is feeling called out right now, take a breath. That feeling? That's not shame. That's recognition. It's your body whispering, *Yes. This is me.*

And here's what I want you to know: **Having emotional buttons doesn't mean you're unstable. Being triggered doesn't mean you're overreacting. Feeling *too* sensitive isn't a weakness - it's information.**

You're not broken. You're human. You've simply lived long enough to absorb messages, patterns, and survival strategies that helped you get by—and now, they're no longer serving you.

Let's be real. Most of us weren't taught how to regulate emotions. We were taught how to hide them. Apologize for them. Make other people comfortable with them. Or better yet, just not have them at all.

You may have been praised for being *easygoing* when you were actually dissociating. You may have been called *strong* when you were emotionally shut down. You may have been labeled *dramatic* when you were simply expressing truth no one else wanted to deal with.

So if your buttons are close to the surface, of course, they are. You've been living in a world that treats emotional honesty like a threat. That's why this work is so powerful. Because once you name what's happening inside you, you stop internalizing it as a character flaw. You start seeing it as a signal. A story. A thread you can trace, learn from, and finally, let go of.

The goal isn't to become emotionless. It's to become *self-led.*

You get to feel things. You just don't have to be *driven* by those feelings anymore. You get to have buttons. You just don't have to let anyone else control the panel.

Self-Reflection: Mapping the Pattern

Take a few quiet minutes to explore what's rising for you. This isn't about judgment. It's about awareness. You're simply noticing.

1. What's one emotional button you now recognize in yourself? Give it a name (e.g., rejection, control, not being heard).

2. When did you first remember feeling this way? You don't need a perfect memory—just let your body tell you the truth. What's the earliest time you can recall this feeling showing up?

3. Who tends to push this button now? What dynamic, tone, or relationship seems to activate this feeling most often?

4. What's your usual reaction when this button gets pushed? Do you shut down, get angry, over-explain, retreat, or overfunction? Just notice your pattern.

5. What might it feel like if that button didn't control your response? Imagine that the button is still there, but it's no longer wired to an alarm. What shifts in your body? In your relationships? In your peace?

You don't have to fix anything yet. This is simply a *button awareness check-in.* Just witnessing your patterns is powerful. Awareness *is* the first unbothered act.

In the next chapter, we're going to get even more personal. You'll start identifying your *specific* buttons—what they are, where they came from, and how they keep showing up in your life.

You're going to get clear. And that clarity? It's going to become your compass. Because you can't disconnect a button you haven't named. You can't change what you're unwilling to witness. And once you start noticing your buttons, you begin rewiring your future.

Try This Toolkit

Here's how to start mapping your emotional wiring.

Journal Prompt

When was the first time you remember feeling like your *no* didn't matter? What did you learn from that moment about your own boundaries?

What's My Most Sensitive Button?

Think of a time when someone upset you more than expected. What were they really touching?

Who Wired It In?

Was it a parent, teacher, boss, ex, or society itself?

When Does It Get Pressed Most Often?

Note the patterns: Social media? At work? Around your family?

2-Minute Mindset Reframe
Boundaries aren't walls; they're doors with locks that you control. Saying no doesn't shut people out—it simply invites in healthier interactions.

Sensory Reset
Try the *5-4-3-2-1* grounding exercise.

- Name 5 things you can see

- 4 things you can touch

- 3 things you can hear

- 2 things you can smell

- 1 thing you can taste

Let your body come back to the present moment before making any decision about what to allow or deny.

Power Statement:
My boundaries are an act of self-respect, not rejection.

Awareness is the greatest agent for change.

— Eckhart Tolle

CHAPTER 3

IDENTIFYING YOUR PERSONAL BUTTONS

You snap. Again. Even though you promised yourself you wouldn't. Your heart's racing, your face is hot, and that voice in your head screams, *Why did I let them get to me again?* Now imagine the same moment, only this time, you pause, breathe, and respond with clarity. That's how you rewire.

Up until now, we've been laying the foundation, talking about what emotional buttons are, where they come from, and how they impact your nervous system. But now we shift. This is where you go from awareness to action.

By now, you've learned what defines emotional buttons, how they're installed, and why they get activated. But now it's time to go deeper. It's time you started naming your own buttons. Not someone else's. Not your mom's, not your partner's, not your coworker's. **Yours.**

Before you can disconnect your buttons, you have to know what they are. I wish this were as simple as a checklist. But emotional buttons are sneaky. They often show up when you least expect it, during a conversation that felt harmless, a text message you can't stop rereading, a comment that sits in your chest for hours. These aren't random. They're clues.

It's about *understanding* yourself. Because once you can name your buttons, you can stop letting them run the show.

It's Not Just Self-Awareness. It's Self-Protection.

Identifying your emotional buttons isn't about overanalyzing yourself or giving yourself more to fix. It's about reclaiming your power. When you know what sets you off, and why, it doesn't control you anymore. You stop bracing. You stop spiraling. You start responding. That's not weakness. That's emotional leadership. It's protection for you and those around you.

Emotional buttons live at the intersection of pain, memory, and meaning. They form in response to unmet needs, unresolved trauma, or conditioned responses. And they almost always show up when you feel any of the following.

- Misunderstood

- Unseen

- Rejected

- Unloved

- Out of control

You might not consciously *think* those things in the moment, but your body reacts like it's true. That's how you know a button's been pushed.

Here's what that might look like:

- You're in a meeting and someone talks over you. You smile and stay quiet, but spend the rest of the day ruminating and doubting yourself.

- Your partner forgets something important. Instead of expressing disappointment, you shut down and convince yourself it's not worth bringing up.

- A friend cancels plans, and you immediately

wonder if you're too much, not enough, or just being avoided.

These are button moments. They're not about what happened. They're about what it *meant* to you. The most common mistake people make is trying to push these feelings away. This sounds like: *It's not a big deal.* Or, *I'm being dramatic.* Or even, *I should be over this by now.* But your body doesn't care about logic. It cares about survival. And if it recognizes something familiar, it reacts fast.

When My Control Button Hijacked the Entire Afternoon

It started with a text. Just a simple, innocent question: *Hey, did you follow up with that client who didn't reschedule last week?*

That was it. No exclamation points. No passive-aggression. Just a basic logistical check-in. But my body? You'd have thought someone pulled the fire alarm inside my nervous system.

I was sitting in my office at the wellness center, already neck-deep in what I call *emotional triage.* You know the days, the printer won't print, a client cancels last minute, someone forgot to load the halotherapy salt chamber, and you're somehow running reception, acting as a crisis counselor, business strategist, and janitor all before lunch.

And then *that* text hit. Immediately, my stomach dropped. Not dramatically, like in a movie. More like a slow, hot flip. My jaw tightened. My shoulders, which were already creeping toward my ears, locked into a full-blown stress shrug. I couldn't even take a breath deep enough to land in my diaphragm. Just shallow, quick gulps like I was prepping for a silent meltdown.

And here's the thing, I *had* followed up with the client. I had even sent a polite *just checking in* email. But that wasn't the point. The point was that my **control** button got smashed. And it set off the **failure** button right behind it, like emotional dominoes falling in my nervous system.

The voice in my head wasn't saying, *Oh, let me check on that.* It was saying, *You should've done more. You're dropping the ball. Everyone's going to think you don't have it together. See? This is why you can't take your foot off the gas.*

It's wild how quickly the internal spiral can start over something so small. But the truth is, it wasn't small to my system. It was *familiar*. It hit an old pattern, one built on the belief that if I don't manage every detail, something will break, and I will be blamed. That belief didn't start at the wellness center. It started decades ago, when I learned that being in control made me feel safe, competent, and valuable. It made me lovable. Or at least... *tolerable*.

So even though I was sitting in a modern, peaceful office with an aromatherapy diffuser blasting essential oils and a Himalayan salt lamp glowing in the corner, my body was back in survival mode. Because that's what happens when emotional buttons get pushed: your nervous system doesn't check the calendar. It just reacts.

And look, I can laugh about it now. Because let's be honest, there was nothing noble about me frantically scanning my inbox with one hand while stress-eating an expired KIND bar with the other. But in the moment? It felt *urgent*. Existential, even.

That one message triggered every part of me that still believes, *You don't get to drop the ball. You don't get to rest–because if something falls through the cracks, it's your fault. And if it's your fault...you're not enough.* That's the script. That's the wiring. That's the button.

Here's what I know now. The button wasn't the problem. The story it was wired to, that's what needed my attention. So I took a breath. I rolled my shoulders back down from my ears. I replied to the text with, *Yes! I followed up with them last week, but there has been no response yet.*

And that was it. No extra proof. No over-explaining. No apology tour. Just the facts. And even though it felt small, it was actually *huge.* Because in that moment, I didn't let the button take the wheel. I saw it. I named it. And I chose not to let it run the show. That's what doing the work looks like, not perfection, but *pattern recognition with a pause button.*

Why This Matters

You might know you feel anxious when your partner pulls away or that you get defensive when someone questions your choices, but do you know *why?*

Every emotional button is wired to something. A belief. A fear. A memory. A role you've been playing for far too long. And you can't unplug a button you haven't named.

That's what we're doing here. Getting specific. Getting honest. Getting free.

Thanks to **neuroplasticity,** the brain's remarkable ability to adapt, rewire, and form new neural connections, we're not confined to our past emotional patterns or knee-jerk reactions. Every time we choose a different response, practice a calming technique, or interrupt a negative thought loop, we're literally reshaping our brain's circuitry. Research shows that with consistent practice, these new pathways can become dominant, making healthier, more regulated responses not only possible but automatic over time. In short, we're not stuck; we're biologically equipped for emotional transformation.

In order to make these changes, you need key tools. So, I want you to practice what I call **The Rewire Ritual.** I will go into more detail in the next few sections, but for now, just remember these three steps.

- **Pause the Pattern** – Interrupt the automatic reaction with a deep breath or grounding technique.

- **Name the Button** – Call out what's being activated: *This is my abandonment wound,* or *This is my performance trigger.*

- **Choose a New Response** – Visualize your desired behavior or say a calming phrase aloud.

Pause. Name. Choose. Seems simple, doesn't it? Let's break these down even more.

What to Look For - Pause

Emotional buttons tend to show up in patterns. You'll often see the same reaction triggered by different people, situations, or even phrases. It's like your nervous system keeps getting the same email from different senders.

Before we dig deeper, take a moment to answer these questions with your gut, no overthinking required.

- **What situation do you dread, even when there's no immediate danger?** (e.g., being called into a meeting, receiving a vague *we need to talk* text)

- **Who in your life makes you feel like you're always walking on eggshells?** Why do you think that is?

- **What do you often feel the need to over-explain or defend?** When does it feel unsafe to just say no?

- **What's a criticism or comment that instantly triggers shame, even if you know it's not true?** What button is that pressing?

- **What's one pattern you keep repeating in different relationships (romantic, family, work)?** What reaction keeps showing up?

So how do you identify your personal buttons? You start with the reaction. Think about the last time your body went into overdrive, your heart raced, your stomach dropped, you shut down, or exploded. Trace it back. What were you feeling before the reaction? Then ask yourself, *What story did I tell myself in that moment? What wound did this trigger? Where have I felt this before?*

These questions can feel uncomfortable. But they're gold. They help you map your internal wiring and start making conscious choices instead of being emotionally hijacked.

That story you keep telling yourself, whether it's, *I'm not safe. I'm not good enough,* or *they're going to leave,* is usually tied to a button. If you want to change your reactions, you have to interrupt the loop before it hijacks your voice, your mood, or your peace. No pause? No power. When you skip the pause, you default to the same old survival script.

Take Inventory: Which Buttons Belong to You? - Name

By now, you've been introduced to some of the most common emotional triggers, and chances are, a few of them hit close to home. The next step is to turn inward and ask yourself: *Which ones feel the most familiar in my life?*

Below is a recap of the emotional buttons we've explored and a few new ones that may hit home for you. You don't need to rank them. You don't need to justify why they exist. You're simply noticing what lights up in your body, your memory, or your relationships when you read them.

- **Rejection:** Feeling unwanted, unchosen, or ignored

- **Abandonment:** The fear that people will leave when you need them most

- **Control:** Needing things to go *just right* in order to feel safe

- **Criticism:** Feeling flawed, exposed, or not good enough

- **Failure:** Believing that mistakes make you unworthy or unlovable

- **Silencing:** Believing your voice, needs, or emotions are *too much*

- **Guilt:** Feeling overly responsible for how others feel or behave

- **Injustice:** Feeling activated when things feel unfair or when people manipulate the rules to benefit themselves

There's no right or wrong here. Some of these may overlap. Some might feel deeply embedded, while others show up only in certain contexts. This is your emotional blueprint, and knowing it is power.

Take a moment to highlight or write down your top three to five buttons. You don't have to have all the answers right now. You just need to start listening to what your body, your reactions, and your history are trying to tell you.

Identifying Example: The Good Girl Glitch

Sometimes we don't even realize the button is there until resentment creeps in. Melanie has been praised her whole life for being sweet, agreeable, and easygoing. Her report cards always said *a joy to have in class*, and no one ever had a complaint–except Melanie herself, quietly resenting every yes she said when she meant no. As an adult, she finds it nearly impossible to express frustration without guilt. That *Good Girl* button got installed early. And now? It's the reason she dreads conflict, avoids boundaries, and feels responsible for everyone's feelings but her own.

Button Mapping: What Pushes Me, and Why?

Now, let's start a personal inventory. Use this space to get honest about where your buttons show up and what they're connected to.

- **Step 1: Identify the Button**

What's the emotional reaction you experience most often?

- **Step 2: Name the Trigger**

Who or what tends to push that button?

- **Step 3: Track the Pattern**

When did this start? What's the earliest memory or relationship where this showed up?

- **Step 4: Notice the Story**

What does that moment *say* to you? What fear or belief rises up?

- **Step 5: Notice Your Response**

What do you typically do when that button gets pushed? Do you freeze? Fawn? Fight? Numb out?

You might journal through just one button today, or come back and fill this in over time. The point is clarity. You can't claim your power if you don't know where it's leaking.

Noticing Your Physical Cues

When Your Body Flags a Button

Sometimes, your body knows before your brain catches up. Your shoulders tense. Your jaw locks. Your stomach flips. You may not even have words for it yet, but your nervous system is already sounding the alarm. It's like your body is waving a little red flag, whispering, *Hey, something familiar is happening.*

You might notice your breathing goes shallow, like your chest can't quite expand. A tight knot forms in your stomach, and your heart begins to race, even though there's no clear danger in sight. You feel tension building in your neck or your back, like you're carrying something heavy you can't quite name. Sometimes, it shows up as a sudden urge to shut down, fix something immediately, or escape the moment altogether. You might feel flushed, shaky, jittery, or completely on edge for reasons that don't seem to match the moment.

This isn't random. It's your body remembering. And it's doing its best to protect you, the only way it knows how, by alerting you to what it perceives as a threat. But just because your body reacts doesn't mean you have to follow that reaction.

One of the most powerful things you can do in those moments is pause—not to suppress the feeling, but to witness it.

Ask yourself gently, ***What just happened? What story am I telling myself right now?***

You don't have to judge the story. You don't even have to fix it yet. Just name it. Because every time you bring awareness to that moment, without shame, without spiraling, you create a tiny pocket of space where your truth gets to breathe. And that space? That's where freedom starts.

Real-Life Examples

In a relationship:
You ask for space, and your partner sighs and says, *You're always so sensitive.*

- Button: Silencing

- Response: You retreat and start second-guessing your needs.

At work:
You're left out of a decision you should've been part of.

- Button: Rejection

- Response: You pretend not to care but stew all day.

As a parent:
Your child has a meltdown in public, and someone gives you a look.

- Button: Criticism or Shame

- Response: You overcorrect or shut down emotionally.

Each of these moments isn't just about what's happening. They're about what that moment *activates* inside you. When you start recognizing the button instead of reacting to it, that's when everything begins to shift.

Before You Move On...

Take a few minutes to reflect on what came up for you in this chapter.

Which three to five emotional buttons feel most present in your life right now?

Where do you feel them most - relationships, work, parenting, or somewhere else?

What do you want to do differently the next time one of them gets pushed?

Taking Back Your Story - Choose

This isn't about control. It's about awareness. And awareness is your access point to becoming unbothered.

Let me remind you of something important, especially if you're the type who feels like once you start healing, you have to *do it all, fix it all, and get it perfect* right away (hi, fellow overachievers).

You don't have to fix it all right now. In fact, trying to rush this process can become its own kind of button. That *I need to figure it all out immediately* voice? It's just another story rooted in pressure, perfectionism, and old survival instincts.

This chapter isn't about solving every trigger in one sitting. It's about naming what's true. And that's more than enough.

The goal isn't to become someone who never reacts, never feels, or never gets thrown off by life. The goal is *clarity*. Clarity gives you choices. It gives you language. It gives you space between the button being pushed and the story being believed.

Every button you name is one step closer to disconnecting it. Not in a dramatic, overnight, *I've transcended all human emotion,* kind of way, but in a quiet, consistent, *I see what's happening and I don't have to live from that place anymore,* kind of way. That's what freedom actually looks like.

So if all you do today is circle three buttons that feel real for you, or write one sentence that helps you understand why that old criticism still stings, you're doing the work. You're breaking cycles. You're beginning again. And that? That's everything.

Try This Toolkit

Journal Prompt

What boundary have you been afraid to set and why? Whose reaction are you most worried about?

2-Minute Mindset Reframe

You're not too much for naming your needs. You're just no longer shrinking to fit other people's comfort zones.

Sensory Reset

Place one hand on your chest and the other on your stomach. Close your eyes and take three slow, intentional breaths. With each inhale, silently say: *I am allowed.* With each exhale: *To take up space.*

Power Statement

I honor what I need, even when it's inconvenient for others.

Not everything that provokes you deserves a response.

— Unknown

CHAPTER 4
WHY DO PEOPLE PUSH BUTTONS?

One of the most exhausting parts of emotional growth is realizing that some people *like* getting a reaction out of you. Others don't mean to, but they do it anyway. And some do it so often, you start to wonder if you're the problem. People push buttons for different reasons—and most of them have **nothing to do with you**.

Sometimes they're testing your limits. Sometimes they're projecting their own shame. Sometimes they're modeling behavior they saw growing up. And sometimes... they're just reacting from their own unhealed pain.

But your reaction? That's what trains them. When someone sees that a certain phrase, tone, or behavior sends you spiraling, and they want power over you, *they'll use it again.*

You weren't born with your buttons exposed. People found them. Pressed them. Repeatedly. Until you learned to flinch, to react, to defend. But why do they push? The answer says more about *them* than it ever did about you.

Up until now, we've been focused on *your* buttons, where they came from, how they were wired in, and how to start naming them with compassion instead of shame. But now it's time to flip the lens. Because sometimes, the healing doesn't come from just understanding *why you react;* it comes from realizing *why someone might be provoking you in the first place.*

And that's where we start shifting from self-blame to strategic clarity. You see, button-pushers are everywhere. Sometimes they're subtle. Sometimes they're loud. Sometimes they have no idea they're doing it—and other times, they've perfected the art of getting under your skin like it's their part-time job.

So the question becomes, ***Why do people push buttons?*** And what do they gain from keeping you reactive, off balance, or self-doubting? Let's talk about it.

The Four Button-Pusher Archetypes

Over the years, I have noticed a pattern in how button-pushers show up in relationships. While this list might not cover all of the button-pushers in your life, I believe most will fall into one of these four categories. The purpose of this list is not to heap shame on these people by labeling them. It's meant to help you identify how they push buttons and why, so that you can be proactive. The more you understand your button-pusher's mindset, the better you become at responding, or not, to their methods.

The Controller

- Needs to manage others to feel safe.

Controlling people often thrive on **emotional predictability**. If they know exactly how you'll react, they feel powerful. If you always defend yourself, cry, over-explain, or shut down, they can manipulate the situation to their benefit.

The Mirror

- Projects their own shame or insecurity onto others.

These individuals don't necessarily *mean* to hurt you, but they **react to the discomfort of seeing in you what they haven't faced in themselves**. Your calmness might highlight their chaos. Your healing might mirror their avoidance. Your confidence might expose their insecurity.

The Manipulator

- Seeks power or emotional chaos to stay in control.

This is the person who has studied your patterns and uses them strategically. They know what will guilt you, silence you, or make you question yourself, and they **use that knowledge to control your reactions**. They weaponize your empathy. Shift blame subtly. Mix praise and criticism to keep you chasing validation. What makes this archetype dangerous is its ability to make you feel like *you're the problem*, while they maintain power over your emotional state. Their goal isn't connection, it's **control disguised as concern**.

The Wounded

- Reenacts unhealed trauma—they aren't trying to hurt you..

Not all button-pushers are manipulative. Some are just unaware. They've never done the work to explore their own emotional patterns, and so they operate on autopilot, creating chaos wherever they go.

Keep these archetypes in mind as we go deeper into what makes button-pushers tick. It will help you quickly identify these people in your life. Button-pushers rarely want your growth. They want their own comfort, even if it costs you peace. They push to provoke, to control, to manipulate. Not because of who you are, but because of what they need. You are not a remote control. Just because someone pushes doesn't mean you have to react.

Archetype Example: After All I've Done For You

Some button-pushers operate from a place of emotional debt. You owe them—forever. Whenever Devon tries to say no to his mother, she sighs heavily and reminds him of all the sacrifices she's made. *I gave up everything for you,* she'll say. *Is it too much to ask for a little help?* Suddenly, Devon's clear boundary feels like betrayal. This guilt-button wasn't born overnight—it was crafted slowly, through years of emotional scorekeeping. People like Devon's mom may not even see it as manipulation, but for the person on the receiving end, it's exhausting and emotionally entangling.

When Pushing Your Button Gives Them Power

Sometimes people push buttons because they want control. Sometimes they want attention, validation, or dominance. And sometimes? They want a distraction from the chaos inside themselves.

When someone lacks emotional regulation, pushing your buttons becomes a shortcut. Instead of dealing with their own discomfort, they use *you* to absorb it. They provoke you because your reaction gives them a sense of power they don't know how to access on their own.

Let's say your coworker constantly questions your decisions in meetings. That button she's pressing, it's not about your competence. It's about her fear of being overlooked. She pushes your 'imposter syndrome' button to soothe her own. She's the **Mirror** archetype.

Let me be clear: not all button-pushers are villains. Some of them are scared. Some are insecure. Some are emotionally immature. Some are just operating on autopilot, running trauma scripts they never questioned.

But just because we can understand it doesn't mean we have to accept it.

It's Not About You - It's About What They Need to Feel

Let's say that louder for the people in the back. **It's not about you. It's about what they need to feel.**

When someone criticizes you out of nowhere, what are they actually trying to feel? Maybe they want to feel superior, right, in control, or emotionally *above* you. When someone guilt-trips you, they're not seeking connection; they're seeking *compliance*.

This is what I call emotional outsourcing. They don't want to process their feelings, so they hand them to you. They push your button, and boom, now *you're* the one scrambling, apologizing, reacting, explaining.

Now *they* feel better. And *you* feel exhausted. And you start thinking, *What's wrong with me? Why am I so triggered by this?* But that's the wrong question.

The right question is, ***Why are they so invested in getting a reaction from me?***

The Day I Didn't Take the Bait

I remember a moment, not all that long ago, when someone I used to be close to reached out to *check in*. I hadn't heard from her in a while, and to be honest, I wasn't surprised. Our friendship had slowly unraveled after I started creating clearer boundaries in my personal life, stepping back from always being the fixer, the listener, the one available at all hours.

At first, the message seemed innocent enough. She asked how I was doing. She said she missed me. But woven into the words were those little barbs I'd come to recognize. Just sharp enough to sting, but soft enough to make me question whether I was imagining it.

I figured I'd hear from you eventually... I know you've been busy doing your own thing.

There it was: the guilt hook. Old me would've scrambled to explain. To apologize for not calling. To prove that I still cared, still showed up, still hadn't become *too much*, or *too full of myself*, or whatever story she was spinning.

But this time? I paused.

I felt the pull, that familiar internal tug to rescue the moment and smooth it over. My chest got tight. My heart sped up just a bit. But then I exhaled and reminded myself: *This is a button. It's being pushed. But I don't have to press back.*

I didn't ignore her. I didn't clap back. I simply responded with warmth and boundaries.

It's been a full season for sure. I hope you're doing well, too.

No justification. No apology. No spiral. Just... neutrality. And a clean return to my own peace. And you know what happened? She never replied.

That used to devastate me. Now? It confirms what I suspected: this wasn't about reconnecting. It was about *testing*. Seeing if the old version of me would still show up, the one who dropped everything to make other people comfortable, even if it cost me my mental health.

She pushed a button. But this time, there was no emotional doorbell wired to it. No guilt. No fawning. No frantic need to be seen as *good*. I saw it for what it was: a moment of manipulation dressed in nostalgia. And for once, I chose not to participate.

That's the power of naming your buttons and understanding the game. You stop playing by their rules. You stop handing out access to people who only show up when they want something from you.

Emotional Baiting: It's Not a Conversation—It's a Trap

Let's talk about one of the most subtle, confusing forms of button-pushing: **emotional baiting.**

This one is sneaky. It often shows up dressed like vulnerability or connection, but the minute you respond, you realize you've been set up. The goal wasn't dialogue. It wasn't closeness. It was *reaction.*

Emotional baiting is when someone says or does something to provoke a response, not because they want to understand you or grow together, but because they want *power.* And if they can't feel powerful through honesty or accountability, they'll get it by pulling you out of alignment.

Here's how the baiting cycle usually plays out.

They poke you - subtly or directly.

- *Wow, you've really changed.*

- *I guess I'm just too much for you now.*

- *I didn't want to say anything, but...*

They wait for you to react - guilt, defensiveness, over-explaining.

- Your button gets pushed.

- Your nervous system lights up.

- You respond.

They flip it on you - suddenly *you're* the one with the problem.

- *See? I can't say anything around you.*

- *You're so sensitive.*

- *This is why I don't bring things up.*

Sound familiar?

This tactic is incredibly common in emotionally manipulative relationships, and it's often rooted in *insecurity and avoidance*. Instead of owning their own discomfort or asking for what they really need, the baiter pushes your buttons just enough to shift the emotional spotlight onto *you*. **Because if you're the one reacting, *they* don't have to.**

What Makes Baiting So Effective?

It works because it taps into your empathy. Your desire to be understood. Your habit of over-explaining to prove you're *not the bad guy.* The baiter relies on your sensitivity and uses it against you. And if you grew up learning that your role is to de-escalate, make peace, or emotionally manage others, baiting can pull you into the same old roles without even realizing it.

So What Do You Do Instead?

You pause. You feel the button get pushed. And you *don't take the bait.*

You might say, *I'm not available for guilt today,* or, *Let me know if there's something you actually want to talk through.* One of the most effective responses comes in the form of curious observation. *That sounded like a dig. Was it?* Or sometimes, silence is your strongest response.

You don't have to justify your boundaries. You don't have to clarify your intentions over and over. You don't have to make it okay for them. Just because someone tosses you emotional bait doesn't mean you have to bite.

Button Pushing in the Wild: Where It Shows Up

You've probably seen this before, but maybe you didn't have language for it. Here's how button-pushing plays out across different dynamics.

In Families

Your mother makes a backhanded comment about your parenting. *Oh, I never let you watch that much TV growing up. But, I mean, do what works for you.* Translation: She's pushing your *criticism* button and masking it as concern.

Your adult sibling reminds you for the forty-seventh time that you *never call*. Guilt button, activated.

In Romantic Relationships

Your partner gives you the silent treatment instead of expressing disappointment directly. This hits the *abandonment* and *control* buttons all at once.

They also might say things like, *You're just overreacting again.* That's *gaslighting* disguised as feedback. They're trying to shut down the conversation and shift the blame onto your emotions.

In Friendships

A friend jokes, *Wow, ever since you started working on your boundaries, you've gotten kinda intense.* **Sarcasm is the lazy person's weapon of choice.** That's a *silencing* button with a punchline.

Another classic, *It must be nice to have so much free time.* Translation: They feel bitter and want you to feel guilty about enjoying your life.

At Work

A colleague CCs your boss on an email about a minor mistake. That's about control and power. Not correction or *performance.* They want your reaction to reinforce their importance.

The Power Dynamics at Play

Let's go a layer deeper. Button-pushing isn't just personal, it's often *positional.* People in perceived authority (parents, bosses, mentors) are more likely to push buttons to maintain power.

Why? Because if you're confused, apologetic, or always on the defense, you're easier to manage. You're less likely to challenge the status quo. You're more likely to stay small.

This is especially true in systems where emotional needs were ignored or weaponized. In families with unspoken roles, in workplaces with toxic leadership, in relationships with lopsided emotional labor. Button-pushing is a tactic. Sometimes conscious. Sometimes conditioned. But always about control.

Emotional Enmeshment: When They Can't Tell Where They End and You Begin

This one's subtle, but *so* common. Enmeshment happens when someone believes your feelings are their responsibility or vice versa. There are no boundaries, no space. Just emotional fusion.

They say things like, *I just can't be okay if you're upset with me.* Or the classic, *After everything I've done for you...* And the blame-shifting standby, *Why didn't you tell me how you were feeling sooner?*

It can feel like love or closeness, but it's not. It's *entanglement.* And when someone is enmeshed with you, your independence threatens them. So they push buttons to reestablish connection. Not healthy connection. But control disguised as closeness.

And sometimes, enmeshment doesn't look explosive or aggressive. It shows up in soft guilt. In subtle pressure. It's the kind of emotional bait that makes you question your boundaries, not because someone says *you're wrong*, but because they act like *you're hurtful* for having any in the first place.

Let me show you what I mean.

The *Martyr* Move

A few years ago, I was deep in a season of recovery, physically, emotionally, and energetically. I was learning to prioritize rest, space, and silence. I had *finally* given myself permission to not be on call for everyone else's emotional needs 24/7.

And that's when the bait showed up. Family edition.

It came in the form of a group text. A relative was organizing a last-minute gathering. No real agenda, just: *We thought it would be nice to see everyone.* I politely declined. I had already committed to rest that weekend, and I knew

I wouldn't have the capacity to hold space for extended small talk and subtle family tension.

Their response, *It's okay, I get it. Everyone's busy. We just wanted to keep the tradition going, but I guess those days are gone now.*

That sentence? Master-level emotional bait. It wasn't a direct attack. It was a soft jab. Wrapped in disappointment, dipped in martyrdom, and served with a side of guilt. The kind that makes you wonder if you're being selfish... even when you know you're just being *well*.

For a split second, the urge to explain myself roared up. I thought, *Should I say more? Should I offer to stop by just for an hour? Should I clarify that I do care about family?*

But I caught it. That's the trap. That's the hook. And so, I replied simply, *Thanks for understanding. I hope it's a great time with everyone.*

And then I let it go. Did it feel a little uncomfortable? Yes. Did it eat at me for the rest of the day? Absolutely not. Because I knew what was happening, and I refused to confuse guilt with obligation.

It would be easy to get angry at moments like that. And honestly, sometimes anger is valid. But here's the thing:

not every button-pusher is scheming or malicious. A lot of the time, they're just acting out old patterns, using emotional habits they don't even realize are harmful, because no one ever taught them a different way.

When Button-Pushers Don't Even Know They're Doing It

Just because someone pushes your buttons doesn't always mean they're calculating or cruel. Sometimes, they're running old emotional programs they don't even realize are still operating. They might guilt-trip because that's how they were raised. They might criticize because that's how they motivate themselves. They might shut down because no one ever taught them how to handle discomfort. **It's not personal, it's patterned.** And recognizing that can help you stop taking the bait while still holding your boundaries with compassion and clarity.

Let's give grace where it's due. Not all button-pushers are malicious manipulators. Some are just emotionally underdeveloped. They've been surviving with these behaviors for so long, they don't even recognize them as dysfunctional. They guilt-trip because that's how their mom got what she wanted. They shut down because no one ever taught them how to self-regulate.

You're not responsible for their growth. But recognizing their patterns helps you stop personalizing them.

The Button-Pusher's Playbook

Let's call out a few greatest hits. These are common button-pushing scripts, some obvious, some subtle. You've probably heard them. You've probably brushed them off. Maybe you've even defended the person who said them, telling yourself, *They didn't mean it like that.* But trust me: your body caught it, even if your brain tried to reason it away. These lines are designed, consciously or not, to make you doubt yourself, over-explain, or fall back into old patterns. And the faster you can spot them, the faster you can stay rooted in your own truth instead of getting pulled into someone else's emotional storm.

You're being dramatic.

→ Translation: *Let me invalidate your emotional truth so I don't have to engage with it.*

You've changed.

→ Translation: *You're not giving me the same unbothered access you used to.*

Wow, must be nice.

→ Translation: *I'm bitter, but I don't want to own that, so I'll disguise it as shade.*

I guess I just won't say anything next time.

→ Translation: *I want to make you responsible for my silence.*

The more familiar you become with these scripts, the less they stick. You can still hear them, but they lose their grip.

Understanding Is Not Excusing

Let me be clear. **Understanding why someone pushes your buttons is not the same as excusing it.** We're not doing this to justify bad behavior. We're doing this so you can stop internalizing it.

You can have compassion for someone's woundedness and still say, *This behavior is not okay.* You can understand their story without writing yourself into it. This chapter is about taking your power back, not by fighting, not by fixing, but by *seeing clearly.*

Because the moment you stop personalizing their behavior? That's the moment you become unbothered.

Take It Off Your Shoulders

Before we close this chapter, take a few minutes to check in with yourself.

- Who in your life has a pattern of pushing your buttons?

- What do they gain from your reaction?

- What story do you tell yourself when it happens?

- And what would shift if you stopped making it your job to manage their behavior?

Awareness doesn't make you cold. It makes you see things clearly. And clarity is where your power lives. Every time you see the button-pusher for who they are, not who they convince you to be, you reclaim your power. You don't have to play the role they're scripting. You can rewrite the scene.

Try This Toolkit

Journal Prompt

Who in your life tends to trigger the strongest emotional reaction in you? What might they be mirroring back that still needs healing?

2-Minute Mindset Reframe

Button-pushers often reveal the emotional work we haven't finished, not the weaknesses we need to hide. Their behavior says more about *them* than it ever will about *you*.

Sensory Reset

Rinse your hands or face in cool water. As the temperature shifts your nervous system, say out loud: *This is mine. That is theirs.* Repeat until your breath slows and your body feels more grounded.

Power Statement

I refuse to carry what was never mine to hold.

PART II

Building the Unbothered Button

Between stimulus and response there is a space. In that space is our power to choose our response. In our response lies our growth and our freedom.

— Viktor E. Frankl

CHAPTER 5
AWARENESS –
THE FIRST STEP
TO BECOMING
UNBOTHERED

You can't disconnect a button if you don't know it's been pushed. Let's start there. Who taught you that saying 'no' made you selfish? What if you stopped feeling guilty for protecting your peace? You were taught to be nice. Not whole. **That ends now.**

Sometimes we don't even realize we've been emotionally hijacked until it's already happened. Until we're deep in a spiral, mid-snap, or apologizing for something that wasn't even our responsibility. Our nervous system beats our brain to the punch. That's not weakness, it's wiring. And unless we slow it down, that wiring keeps running the show.

Becoming unbothered doesn't happen by accident.

You don't wake up one day magically immune to the guilt trips, emotional landmines, or chaos around you. It starts with one powerful shift: awareness. Awareness is the moment we interrupt that pattern. It's the first real step in becoming unbothered. And make no mistake, it's a skill. It's something you practice, not something you magically possess.

That's it. That's the first step. Not boundaries (yet). Not confrontation. Not silence or walking away. It starts with noticing. Most people try to skip this part because it doesn't feel like *doing something*. But awareness is *everything*. Until you're aware, you're still reacting from habit. Still caught in survival mode. Still operating on emotional autopilot.

What Awareness Actually Means

Identifying the people who consistently push our buttons is only half the equation. True transformation comes when we pair that awareness with a deeper understanding of our own mental and physical state. Button-pushers often activate old emotional wounds, and without noticing it, our bodies respond before our minds even catch up (cue tightened shoulders, shallow breathing, racing thoughts). When we learn to tune into these physiological and psychological cues, we begin to interrupt the automatic stress loop. This self-awareness acts as an internal pause button, allowing us to observe what's happening inside us before reacting to what's happening around us.

Let's get this straight. Awareness isn't about never getting triggered. It's not about pretending you're okay or floating above your feelings like some kind of emotionally enlightened robot.

Awareness is the skill of noticing what's happening inside you without being taken over by it. It's that little voice that says, *Ah. This is familiar.* It's the questioning. *This feels like rejection, but is it really?* It's being attuned enough to recognize, *I want to snap, but what would happen if I just... paused?*

Awareness is the breath between the button getting pushed and the story you attach to it. Without awareness, you're just reacting from habit. With awareness, you get to respond with intention. And that one shift? It changes everything.

The First Big Pause: Choosing Awareness After Recovery

There's something about coming back from a major life disruption, whether it's a health crisis, a loss, or a heartbreak, that sharpens your senses in ways you don't expect.

Brain surgery isn't something you ever imagine will become part of your life story, but for me, it became a defining chapter. I thought the hardest part would be the physical healing. And yes, it was brutal some days. But what caught me off guard was how vulnerable it made my emotional system.

Every little thing felt louder, heavier, sharper. A forgotten text. A misunderstood email. Someone assuming I could just *bounce back* and pick up where I left off. All of it felt personal. All of it hit my emotional buttons in rapid fire.

One afternoon, about a month into recovery, a situation popped up at work. A minor scheduling miscommunication. Normally, it wouldn't have been a big deal. But that day, my body reacted like someone had pulled the fire alarm inside my chest.

Instant panic. No flames, no real danger, just that shrill, urgent noise that makes it feel like everything is falling apart, even when it's not. I could feel it happening. The tightness in my chest, the prickling heat behind my eyes, the thoughts racing. *They think I'm unreliable now, I'm failing, I'm letting everyone down.* Old programming, firing on all cylinders.

I was halfway through typing an apologetic, defensive email when something in me finally said, *Wait. Breathe.* And I did. I took one long, intentional breath. I sat back. I let the wave of shame and urgency pass through me instead of driving me.

And when I re-read the original email, I saw it differently. It wasn't even critical. It wasn't judgmental. It was just... information. A minor fix. A normal human mistake. The story my body wanted to tell, that I was failing, disappointing, crumbling, wasn't the story I had to believe anymore.

Instead of sending a two-paragraph apology, I sent a one-line reply, *Thanks for letting me know. I'll take care of it.* That was it. No spiraling. No over-explaining. No abandoning myself to chase someone else's approval.

And you know what? The world didn't end. No one fired me. No one revoked my credibility.
The only thing that changed was my relationship to my own panic.

That was one of the first times I realized in my bones. Awareness isn't about pretending you're not hurt. It's about noticing the hurt and choosing not to hand over the keys to it.

That single breath didn't just save me from overreacting. It reminded me that even on my hardest days, I still had a choice. And that choice was enough.

You don't need a crisis to learn this. You just need to start paying attention to the moments your body sounds the alarm. And trust yourself enough to pause before you believe the fire.

Button-Spotting in Real Time

Emotional buttons don't come with blinking lights or sirens. They show up quietly, through subtle signals in your body and mind. Here's what to watch for.

- A sudden change in tone, posture, or breathing

- Feeling the urge to explain or defend something that shouldn't need justification

- Thinking, *Oh no, they're mad. What did I do wrong?*

- That tightness in your chest, or the hot flush in your face

- The mental checklist of what you should have said, done, or prevented

These are your internal alerts. When they show up, pause. Ask yourself:

- *What's actually happening right now?*

- *Is this about now, or is this about then?*

- *Am I about to act from alignment... or from anxiety?*

That's awareness. You don't have to do anything yet. You're just noticing.

Awareness in Action: Try These Micro-Practices

Let's get practical. Here are five simple, daily practices you can use to build emotional awareness.

The Three-Breath Reset

When you feel triggered, take three intentional breaths before you respond. Not deep—just deliberate. Inhale, hold for a beat, exhale slower than you inhaled. Repeat.

The One-Word Check-In

Ask yourself throughout the day, *What's one word for how I'm feeling right now?* Not how you should feel. How you actually feel.

Here's an example. At work, your boss skips over you in a meeting.

- One-word check-in = *Dismissed.*

- You notice the sting. But instead of folding into yourself or mentally quitting on the spot, you breathe and stay grounded.

The *Story I'm Telling Myself* Prompt

When something stirs you up, say it out loud. *The story I'm telling myself is...*
It's often not the facts that trigger us. It's the meaning we assign to them.

The Button Tracker

Keep a note on your phone labeled *Buttons.* Each time you notice a reaction that feels disproportionate, jot it down. This isn't about judgment. It's about pattern recognition.

The Post-Reaction Debrief

If you do get activated (because we all do), give yourself five minutes later to reflect. Ask yourself, *What pushed me? What did I need? What could I try next time?*

You don't need to practice them all at once. Start with one. Keep it simple. The goal isn't to control your emotions. It's to stop letting them control you.

The Power of the Pause

Let's be real. Most people move straight from stimulus to spiral. Something happens, and boom, we're in it. Our breath shortens, our thoughts race, our nervous system floods us with urgency. The pause is what breaks that loop.

But if you're like most people, you know this in theory, and still find yourself reacting before you can stop it. Let's talk about what's really at risk when you skip the pause.

What Might Happen If You Skip the Pause

Skipping the pause might not seem like a big deal in the moment. After all, it only takes a few seconds to send the text, fire off the email, raise your voice, or over-apologize... right?

But here's what skipping the pause actually costs you. You overreact to something small, and then spend the rest of the day cleaning up the fallout. You say yes to something you didn't want to do, then resent the person who asked, and yourself for folding. You jump to defend yourself, before realizing the person wasn't even criticizing you. You spiral into over-explaining, over-texting, and over-compensating, only to feel drained, anxious, and emotionally exposed afterward. You agree to a boundary violation because your nervous system convinced you it was safer to please than pause. You lose sleep replaying a moment y ou *could've* handled differently if you had just taken one breath to check in with yourself first.

Sound familiar? That's the hidden cost of skipping the pause. It's not about *getting it wrong*. It's about *losing your center*, handing your emotional power over to someone else's tone, timing, or expectations.

You can't change what someone says or does. But you *can* choose what you do with the moment between their action and your response.

And in that pause? That's where your clarity lives. That's where your power lives. That's where your unbothered button starts to form.

Pause Required: The Replay Loop

Replaying conversations is a trauma loop, not a strategy. After a difficult conversation at work, Vanessa replays every sentence in her mind—what she said, what she didn't say, how they might interpret her tone. By dinner, she's reimagining the whole exchange with a better comeback and mentally drafting an apology just in case. This spiral used to feel like problem-solving, but it's really just anxiety in disguise. Vanessa started practicing a simple grounding trick: naming five things she sees, four she can touch, three she can hear. It interrupts the loop just long enough to rese

t.

Micro-Reactions Are Still Reactions

When we talk about pausing before reacting, most people picture dramatic moments like yelling, crying, throwing their phone across the room. And sure, those are reactions. But the truth is, most of the ways we leak emotional energy aren't explosive. They're subtle. Small. Almost invisible unless you're paying attention.

A clipped *I'm fine* when you're absolutely not fine. A heavy sigh you don't even realize you let out. The slight eye roll you can't quite hide. The one-word text that says more than a whole paragraph ever could. The way your shoulders tense or you go a little quieter, a little colder, even though you keep smiling.

These micro-reactions might seem harmless. And sometimes, they are, if you catch them early and tend to what's underneath. But left unchecked, they slowly erode your sense of clarity. They keep the button wired up and ready for the next trigger.

Because even if you didn't *lose it,* your energy already shifted. Your body already moved into defense. Your heart already closed a little. That's why the pause matters even when you don't feel explosive. That's why noticing matters even when the reaction is small.

You don't need to wait until you're spiraling to choose a different path. You can start by catching the small leaks, one breath, one shift, one moment at a time. And that? That's mastery.

So, how do you catch yourself before the old story takes over? That's where the Pause Protocol comes in.

The Pause Protocol

Step 1: Notice what's happening

Your body will almost always speak first. Pay attention.

Step 2: Name what's familiar

This feels like rejection. This reminds me of my mom's tone. This hits my guilt button.

Step 3: Breathe

No fancy meditation needed. One deep inhale, one longer exhale, one quiet beat of stillness. I like to call this *The First Breath Rule*. If I feel activated, I owe myself at least one full breath before I speak.

Step 4: Choose, don't react

Ask: *What would the unbothered version of me do here?*

You won't always nail it. But every time you pause, even for a breath, you shift your power back into your own hands.

Awareness Isn't Instant - It's a Muscle You Build

Let's be honest: most of us aren't great at this when we first start. We catch ourselves reacting *after* the explosion, *after* the apology text, *after* we're already replaying the conversation in our head and wishing we could do it differently.

That's normal. That's human. That's the messy middle of growth. Awareness isn't about flipping a switch overnight. It's about building emotional muscle memory—one moment, one pause, one breath at a time. Just like physical strength, emotional awareness develops in **layers.**

Basic Level: Noticing physical sensations.
At first, your body will speak before your brain does. You'll notice your jaw tightening, your shoulders creeping toward your ears, your heart racing. You might not know why yet. You just know something is happening.

Mid Level: Catching old emotional narratives starting to activate.

Next, you'll start recognizing the familiar stories that sneak in when your buttons get pushed. Stories like: *I'm being rejected. I'm not good enough. It's my job to fix this.* You won't always stop them immediately. But you'll see them faster than before.

Advanced Level: Choosing your emotional stance before responding.

Over time, awareness becomes proactive. You feel the trigger, name the story, take a breath, and then choose your response from a place of clarity, not fear. You lead yourself, instead of being led by old programming.

It's not about being perfect. It's about catching yourself one second sooner than you would have last year. Progress in awareness isn't measured by how often you feel triggered. It's measured by how quickly you recognize the pattern—and how powerfully you choose to respond.

Every pause, every breath, every *wait a minute* moment is proof that you're building the unbothered button from the inside out. This is growth you *feel* long before anyone else can see it.

Awareness Isn't Passivity

Now, let me be very clear. **Awareness isn't the same as tolerating bad behavior.** This isn't about becoming some zen, spiritualized robot who never gets upset. It doesn't mean you smile politely while someone crosses your boundaries. And it definitely doesn't mean you trade your voice for inner peace.

Awareness simply gives you back the power to *choose* your response instead of being emotionally dragged into one. This is about staying awake in your body and in your truth, even when someone tries to drag you back into your old emotional programming.

You can be fully aware of someone's manipulation and still walk away. You can notice the guilt trip and still say no. You can feel the pull to defend yourself and choose to stay grounded instead. You can feel the sting of criticism without letting it rewrite your worth. **Awareness isn't silence. It's sovereignty.**

Awareness in Action

Not too long ago, I was in a conversation with someone who clearly didn't respect the boundaries I had set. They made a *joking* comment that, in reality, was a dig meant to provoke me. Old me would have either laughed it off to keep the peace or gotten defensive and over-explained why I had a right to set the boundary in the first place.

But awareness gave me a third option. I caught the familiar clench in my stomach.

I noticed the urge to justify myself. And instead of reacting, I paused, breathed, and stayed grounded. I looked them in the eye and said, simply, *"That comment didn't sit well with me. What did you mean by that?"*

No anger. No apology. No emotional labor.

And guess what? They didn't love it. They shifted uncomfortably. But I stayed rooted—and the conversation moved on without me losing my center.

That's what awareness gives you. The ability to address reality *without losing yourself in it.*

You don't ignore disrespect. You don't absorb guilt. You don't explain your worth. You respond—with clarity, with calm, and with full ownership of your energy.

Anchoring Truth - Meekness Isn't Weakness

Our culture often confuses meekness with weakness. But spiritually and energetically, they aren't the same thing at all. Meekness is not about being passive, silent, or weak. It's about having power under control.□

It's about knowing you could lash out, fight back, or retaliate, and choosing, instead, to stay rooted in wisdom, strength, and calm. Not reacting doesn't mean you're weak. It means you're wise enough to protect your peace.

In Matthew 5:5, Jesus says, *Blessed are the meek, for they shall inherit the earth.*

That's not a blessing for the timid. That's a blessing for the disciplined. For those who know how to hold their emotional ground without losing their character.

Real meekness is the ability to stand in full awareness of your power and choose not to let someone else's chaos pull you out of alignment. In other words, awareness isn't passivity. It's the highest form of strength. **Strength isn't in how fast you react. It's in how deeply you choose to stay aligned with your truth.**

Reflection: The Awareness Check-In

Take a few minutes to journal through the following.

- When was the last time I reacted to a button without realizing it?

- What does my body usually do when a button is pushed?

- What *story* do I default to when I feel emotionally activated?

- What would it feel like to pause, breathe, and choose?

You don't need to control everything. You just need to start noticing. Choosing awareness isn't about playing small. It's about standing tall inside yourself before you let anyone else's energy decide who you are.

Once you become aware of your patterns (your triggers, your narratives, your somatic responses), you unlock the power to choose differently. And choice is what separates the bothered from the unbothered. Think about it.

- If someone says something passive-aggressive and you immediately spiral, they own your energy.

- If you feel responsible for everyone else's mood but ignore your own, you've abandoned yourself.

- If you shut down every time you're uncomfortable, your nervous system is still running the show.

But if you can *notice* these moments in real time, without judgment, you start to reclaim power. Lightbulb moment: *Oh, I see what's happening here.* That's the kind of awareness we're building. Noticing without blaming. Observing without spiraling. Becoming the witness instead of the puppet.

Button-pushers thrive on speed. They count on your *automatic* reactions. They want you flustered, unsure, rushing to fix it, spiraling to prove your worth. Awareness breaks the pattern. It introduces a pause. That pause gives you time to breathe, regroup, and remember who you are. **Awareness makes space for intention.** And intention leads to freedom.

Try This Toolkit

Journal Prompt

What emotional reaction are you tired of repeating? What belief might be driving that response?

2-Minute Mindset Reframe

You're not overreacting. You're reacting from a wound. But every time you pause instead of spiraling, you're laying down a new path in your brain. That's not failure. It's rewiring.

Sensory Reset

Use bilateral stimulation. Tap your left and right thighs alternately for one minute while slowly breathing in through your nose and out through your mouth. This simple reset helps calm the emotional brain and bring clarity.

Power Statement

I am not my old reaction. I am becoming someone new, on purpose.

You can't control the first thought that pops into your head—but you can control the second one.

— Unknown

CHAPTER 6
STEP TWO – YOU DON'T HAVE TO BELIEVE EVERYTHING YOU THINK

Your thoughts are not facts. They feel real, they sound convincing, and they can be loud, but that doesn't make them true. Especially when your emotional buttons are being pushed.

When someone triggers you, your brain doesn't calmly assess the situation. It races. It fills in gaps with old stories. It pulls from memory, trauma, insecurity, and fear. And before you even know what's happening, you're running a mental script that was never written by your healthiest self.

When left unchallenged, your thoughts become beliefs, and beliefs drive behavior. You can be fully aware that a button got pushed and still find yourself spiraling if you don't catch the story your brain tries to tell you afterward.

Awareness is essential. But rewiring? That's what changes everything.

This is why the second step to becoming unbothered is learning to **reframe your internal narrative.** You don't have to silence your thoughts. You just have to start questioning them.

Because emotional freedom doesn't come from avoiding triggers. It comes from refusing to live by the same old story every time they show up. This chapter is about catching those moments when your mind tries to drag you down familiar roads, and choosing a new path, even when the old one feels easier.

It's about recognizing the narrative before it becomes your reality. It's about shifting your emotional stance at the root, *in your thinking,* not just in your reacting.

How Thoughts Shape Emotional Reactions

Let's talk about what's really happening when your button gets pushed. It's not just the external situation that sends you spiraling. It's what your mind does *with* the situation. Cognitive Behavioral Therapy (CBT) breaks it down like this:

Situation → *Thought* → *Emotion* → *Behavior*

It's not the situation that creates your emotional storm. It's the *thought* you attach to the situation that triggers the emotional cascade. Here's a quick example.

- **Situation:** Someone criticizes your work.

- **Thought:** *I'm not good enough. They're disappointed in me.*

- **Emotion:** Shame, anxiety, fear.

- **Behavior:** Overexplaining, apologizing, withdrawing, or overworking to *fix it.*

The situation triggered you, but the thought you latched onto *determined the size and intensity* of your emotional response. The good news? If you can catch and shift the thought, you can radically change how you feel and how you act.

You're not trapped by your first thought. You can challenge it—and choose something truer.

Believing the Wrong Story: A Lesson in Rewiring

Not long ago, I caught myself spiraling over something that, on paper, should've been minor. I had emailed a colleague about a collaboration idea I was really excited about. I spent extra time writing it. I made sure I was thoughtful, professional, and clear. Hit send. Felt good about it.

And then... silence. One day. Two days. A week.

Cue the old soundtrack in my mind. Thoughts popped in like, *They're ignoring you,* and *You must've said something wrong.* Left unchecked, those thoughts began to spiral into, *You're too much. You're not enough. You blew it.* And even worse: *They don't want you.*

It didn't matter that I knew better intellectually. Emotionally, my nervous system was playing a greatest-hits album of every rejection wound I thought I had healed. By Day Three, I had half-convinced myself I needed to apologize, for what, I wasn't sure, but surely I had messed something up, right?

Thankfully, somewhere in the middle of all that catastrophizing, I caught myself. I paused. I asked: *Is this thought 100% true?* I challenged: *Is there another way to see this?*

And the more I sat with it, the clearer it became. People get busy. Emails get buried. My worth wasn't hanging in the balance of a single response.

When the reply finally came through, nearly a week later, it was full of apologies. An emergency had come up. They were thrilled about the collaboration idea. They couldn't wait to move forward.

It had *never* been about me. But my brain tried to make it about me because old narratives are sticky.

That experience reminded me why rewiring isn't a one-time fix. It's a daily, deliberate practice of catching the old lies before they rebuild themselves. And most importantly—it reminded me that even when you slip into the wrong story for a minute, you can always, always choose to step back into the truth.

That's the thing about emotional rewiring. It's not about never having old thoughts pop up. It's about learning to catch them before they harden into beliefs. And the tool that makes that possible, the one that will change the entire way you experience emotional triggers, is reframing. Let's talk about how to start.

Reframing the Story

This is where cognitive reframing becomes one of your most powerful tools. **Cognitive reframing** is the practice of intentionally challenging unhelpful thoughts and offering a more balanced or compassionate interpretation. It doesn't mean pretending everything is fine. It means being *willing* to see it differently. Reframing isn't about pretending everything's fine when it's not. It's about telling yourself a version of the story that is *both truer and less destructive* than the one your fear wants you to believe.

It starts with asking a few simple questions.

- *Is this thought 100% true?*

- *Is there another way to see this?*

- *What would a neutral, compassionate version of this story sound like?*

Let's look at an example.

- **Old Story:**
  They didn't text me back. I must have upset them.

I always ruin relationships.

- **Reframe:**
  There could be a hundred reasons someone doesn't text back immediately. It's not evidence that I'm doing something wrong.

See the difference? One story sends you spiraling. The other story lets you stay grounded. You can acknowledge your feelings without feeding them lies. You can hold space for your hurt without giving it a megaphone. Reframing is how you start building new emotional pathways that are rooted in reality, not fear.

At first, these reframes might feel fake. That's normal. You've spent years reinforcing the original thought patterns. But with practice, new thoughts feel more natural, and old ones start to lose their grip. The truth is, most of us have deeply ingrained mental loops we never chose. They were shaped by family dynamics, social messaging, trauma, and repetition. The key is realizing that *you don't have to keep believing them.* You get to rewire your thoughts to support your peace, not sabotage it.

Real World Example

I had a client once who always assumed silence meant punishment. If someone didn't text back, she panicked. If a friend needed space, she spiraled. Together, we traced that pattern back to her childhood, where silence *was* punishment. It made sense. Her brain had been trying to protect her all this time.

Once she saw the origin, she could challenge the belief. She started asking better questions. And eventually, she stopped assuming the worst every time someone went quiet. This is what it means to **become unbothered at the thought level**. You don't shut your thoughts down. You hold them up to the light and ask: *Is this helping me, or hurting me?*

When you start doing this regularly, you become emotionally lighter. You stop feeding fear. You stop reacting to assumptions. You stop giving energy to stories that were never rooted in truth. And you start choosing thoughts that align with the life you're building—not the pain you're healing from.

The Brain Believes What You Tell It

Here's something wild most people don't realize. Your brain's number one job is to keep you alive, not to keep you emotionally accurate. And because of that, your brain will believe almost anything you tell it, especially if it's attached to strong emotion.

If you tell yourself: *I'm a failure,* your brain starts scanning your entire life for evidence to prove you right. If you tell yourself: *No one respects my boundaries,* your brain becomes hyper-alert to every tiny sign of disrespect and starts ignoring the moments when people do honor your boundaries. This is called **confirmation bias,** the psychological tendency to notice and remember information that supports what you already believe, while overlooking anything that challenges it.

Your thoughts build the filters your brain uses to interpret reality. In other words, **what you tell yourself becomes the lens you live through.** That's why reframing your thoughts isn't just a nice idea, it's essential.

When you start telling your brain a new story, one rooted in truth, compassion, and possibility, your brain goes to work finding evidence to support *that*. It's not about lying to yourself.

It's about giving yourself a chance to see the full picture, not just the version your old pain wants you to see.

When you reframe, you're not pretending. You're expanding. You're saying to your mind, *We don't have to live inside the old fears anymore. Let's build something truer, together.* And over time? That becomes your new reality.

That's why the next step isn't just noticing when your brain tells a painful story. It's learning to recognize the specific distortions that keep that story alive, and choosing to rewrite them with truth. If you don't catch the old lies your brain keeps rehearsing, you'll keep living by them, even when they stopped being true a long time ago.

How to Catch Thought Distortions

Most emotional spirals aren't random. They're powered by specific, predictable distortions in your thinking. Learning to spot them is like turning on a light in a dark room—you see the old wiring clearly, and you can start choosing differently.

Catching thought distortions is like casting characters for a bad soap opera you didn't even audition for. Each distortion has its own personality. Here are three of the most common:

Catastrophizing—*The Drama Queen*

Every tiny inconvenience becomes the end of the world. She's always fanning herself dramatically and clutching imaginary pearls.

What this sounds like:

- *This is a disaster.*

- *Everything is ruined.*

- *This one mistake will destroy everything.*

Why it happens:
Your brain tries to predict worst-case scenarios to *protect* you, but ends up flooding you with anxiety.

Reframe:

This feels big, but it's one moment—not my whole story.

Black-and-White Thinking—*The Strict Judge*

Everything is all good or all bad. There's no nuance. No context. Just a very loud gavel slamming down.

What this sounds like:

- *I either succeed completely or I'm a total failure.*

- *If they're upset once, they must hate me.*

Why it happens:
It's easier (and emotionally lazier) for the brain to think in extremes than to sit with nuance.

Reframe:

Both things can be true. I can have a setback and still be making progress.

Personalization—*The Main Character*

Every sideways glance, every delayed text, every weird vibe? Somehow it's all about you.

What this sounds like:

- *They canceled plans—it must mean they don't like me.*

- *Their bad mood must be because of something I did.*

Why it happens:

We center ourselves in situations because it gives us an illusion of control—*if it's about me, maybe I can fix it.*

Reframe:

Other people's emotions are about them, not me. I'm responsible for my behavior, not their mood.

When you start seeing your distortions this way, it gets a little easier to laugh at them. And a lot easier to stop handing them the script to your emotional life. You don't have to kick these characters out. You just don't have to let them run the show.

Catch them. Smile a little. And then choose a different director.

The *Catch It, Challenge It, Change It* Checklist

Now that you know who's been auditioning inside your mind, let's talk about how to catch them before they steal the spotlight and how to rewrite the scene before it plays out the old way.

- **Catch It**
  Notice the thought the moment your body reacts.

- **Challenge It**

Ask: *Is this thought 100% true? Is it helpful? Would I say it to someone I love?*

- **Change It**
  Reframe the thought into something neutral, kind, or empowering, even if it feels awkward at first.

This isn't about toxic positivity. It's about emotional responsibility. It's about choosing not to keep rehearsing narratives that shrink you. You can't stop these characters from showing up. But you can stop handing them the microphone.

Letting Go of Old Stories Is an Act of Courage

Before you start rewriting your emotional patterns, there's something important you need to hear. **You built those old stories for a reason.**

Maybe you learned to expect rejection because it hurt less to assume it was coming. Maybe you believed you had to be perfect to be loved because, somewhere along the way, love started feeling conditional. Maybe you personalized everything because it felt safer to believe you had control, even if it was exhausting.

Those old beliefs weren't flaws. They were survival strategies. They helped you stay connected. They helped you stay prepared. They helped you stay safe.

But survival and thriving aren't the same thing. At some point, what once protected you starts to imprison you. And that's where the work begins, not by blaming your old self, but by honoring who you are and choosing to lead with you in mind.

Rewiring your emotional responses isn't just an act of discipline. It's an act of compassion. It's an act of rescue. It's an act of radical self-loyalty.

You aren't betraying who you were by challenging the old stories. You're keeping the promises your younger self didn't even know how to ask for.

A Permission Slip for the Work Ahead

It's okay if this feels tender. It's okay if you notice resistance, sadness, or even anger rising up.□
It doesn't mean you're failing. It means you're touching something real.

Growth often feels like grief at first. You're not just building new stories. You're honoring the part of you that survived with the old ones.

Take a breath. Give yourself grace. And know this. **You are exactly where you're supposed to be. You're not broken. You're rebuilding.**

One thought at a time. One truth at a time. One act of loyalty to yourself at a time. You're doing it.

This is your reminder: Growth is allowed to feel tender and brave at the same time.

Visualization and Journaling Tools

The Emotional Rewiring Room

Imagine this. Every time you catch an old thought and choose not to feed it, you're redecorating your internal world. You're walking into a new mental room.

Imagine stepping into that room inside your mind. At first, the old echoes might still bounce off the walls. It's familiar, but not in a good way. The walls are lined with old posters of rejection, failure, and fear. The voices of doubt and fear might still rattle around in the corners. You can still hear the echoes from old stories bouncing off the ceiling, saying: *You're not enough. Everyone leaves. You have to be perfect to be loved.*

You didn't decorate this room consciously. It was built little by little, story by story, often without your permission. But now? Now you get to remodel.

Every time you catch a thought distortion and reframe it, you take something off the walls. With every pause, every reframed thought, every moment you choose compassion over catastrophe, you hang up new pictures. You repaint the walls with peace. You build a space that feels like you, not like your old programming. A space that is kinder, truer, and reflects your actual worth, not your old wounds.

At first, the old voices might still echo. That's okay. It doesn't mean you're failing. It just means the remodel is still in progress. Over time, those old sounds get quieter. The space feels lighter. The room becomes a place you want to live in, not one you're trying to escape.

You don't have to tear yourself apart to rebuild your mind. You can rewire it, one breath, one choice, one tiny shift at a time. You get to rewire the room, gently.

Journaling Prompts for Rewiring

You don't have to rebuild everything overnight. But the more you notice, the more you reframe, the more you gently redesign your inner space. Let's start that process now, with a few simple reflection questions to help you step into your new room with clarity.

- *What story did my brain tell me today that I chose to question?*

- *How did I reframe that story into something truer or more compassionate?*

- *How did my body and emotions shift after I changed the story?*

- *What is one thought distortion I catch myself repeating, and what is one truth I can replace it with?*

If you're really looking to go deep on this exercise, here's a bonus prompt for you.

- *If I could decorate one new wall in my Emotional Rewiring Room today, what word, image, or message would I hang there?*

Get descriptive with this one. Make this exercise more playful and imaginative. Allow yourself to feel hopeful about this new space.

As you begin rewiring, don't worry about getting it perfect. These questions are simply invitations to notice, reflect, and keep designing the emotional space you actually want to live in.

You Are the Architect

Rewiring your emotional responses isn't about pretending you don't get hurt anymore. It's not about becoming a perfect version of yourself who never feels doubt or fear again. It's about refusing to build your emotional life on fear. Refusing to let the same old scripts keep you small, scared, or stuck. You're not trying to erase the past. You're building something new alongside it.

You will still feel disappointment. You will still feel anger. You will still feel sadness. But those feelings won't run your life anymore. They won't decide your worth. They won't define your future.

Every time you catch a distorted thought and choose a truer one. Even if you stumble first, you are strengthening the emotional muscles that make you unbothered, unshakable, and free. It won't always feel dramatic. Sometimes it will look like one slow breath instead of a snap. One tiny pause before a text you don't send. One shift from spiraling to staying.

But those tiny moments add up. They build new wiring. They build new stories. They build a new way of living.

You are not at the mercy of your first thought. You are the architect of the story you live from. And every time you catch, challenge, and change an old narrative, you lay another brick on the path to emotional freedom. Keep building. You're closer than you think.

Try This Toolkit

Journal Prompt
What's one boundary you've been avoiding setting because you're afraid of how someone might respond? What would change for you if you set it anyway?

2-Minute Mindset Reframe
Avoiding a boundary to keep the peace often creates a war inside yourself. You don't owe anyone comfort at the cost of your own clarity.

Sensory Reset
Stand tall, feet grounded, and say your boundary out loud—even if no one is there. Feel the vibration in your chest and throat. Let your body remember what it feels like to speak with authority and calm.

Power Statement
My peace matters. I can say it, and still be safe.

Anchoring Truth

As we begin rewiring our emotional responses, it's important to understand that this isn't just about controlling your reactions. It's about *transforming* the way your mind interprets what's happening. **Neuroscience calls it neuroplasticity. Scripture calls it renewal.**

Do not conform to the pattern of this world, but be transformed by the renewing of your mind. **– Romans 12:2**

What we're doing here is more than a mental shift. It's soul work.

Boundaries are the distance at which I can love you and me simultaneously.

— Prentis Hemphil

CHAPTER 7
STEP THREE – SETTING BOUNDARIES

Awareness shows you where the pattern is. Rewiring helps you shift the story inside your mind. But boundaries? **Boundaries are where all that inner work meets the outside world.** Boundaries are how you protect the emotional clarity you're building. They're how you move from emotional defense to empowered leadership over your life.

This is where I remind you, boundaries aren't walls to keep people out. They're bridges that protect connection, respect, and self-trust. When you set a boundary, you're not closing yourself off. You're clearing the path for healthier, more honest relationships.

This is where emotional sovereignty begins. A boundary is a limit or guideline that protects your emotional, mental, physical, or energetic space. It says, *This is what I will allow. This is what I won't. And this is what I need to feel safe and respected.*

This chapter isn't about learning how to *win* against difficult people. It's about learning how to protect your energy, honor your truth, and communicate with clarity, *whether or not* other people like it.

To get this chapter started, I want you to ask yourself...

- *Who taught you that saying 'no' made you selfish?*

- *What if you stopped feeling guilty for protecting your peace?*

You were taught to be nice. Not whole. That programing ends today.

Boundaries Are Proactive Protection, Not Punishment

Let's get something clear from the beginning. **Boundaries are not punishments.** They aren't walls built out of anger. They aren't revenge. They aren't a power move to *teach people a lesson.* They're instructions for how to engage with you. They're not about changing other people. They're about choosing what you'll accept.

Healthy boundaries are proactive self-respect. They're how you care for yourself without apology. They're how you build relationships that are sustainable, not just tolerable.

When you set a boundary, you're saying, *This is how I take care of my energy, my peace, and my purpose.* Not: *This is how I control you.* Definitely not: *This is how I get back at you.*

You're not pushing people away. You're choosing what gets to come close. Remember, boundaries don't box you in. They free you from the chaos of everyone else's expectations.

But let's be honest. For many of us, setting boundaries feels terrifying. Why? Because it risks disapproval. Rejection. Conflict. And for those of us wired for people-pleasing, confrontation feels like danger. But here's what you must remember. **Discomfort is not the same as danger.**

The Emotional Costs of No Boundaries

It's easy to think that setting boundaries is the *hard* part. And yes, learning to speak your truth and hold your ground takes work. But you know what costs even more over time? **Not setting boundaries at all.**

When you live without clear limits, the emotional toll adds up quietly, then all at once. You find yourself saying yes when you mean no. You spend precious time and energy feeling responsible for everyone else's feelings. You find yourself carrying resentment you can't voice without guilt. And eventually, this leaves you feeling exhausted, overstretched, and strangely invisible in your own life.

Setting a boundary might feel uncomfortable, but it's also how you build self-respect. You don't need to be harsh. You don't need to yell. You don't even need to explain yourself at length. You just need to be clear.

Without boundaries, your energy leaks. Your peace erodes. Your self-trust crumbles. And the people around you may not realize it—because, unintentionally, you've taught them that your needs are negotiable.

Please hear me when I say this next part. **Living without boundaries doesn't make you more loving. It makes you more depleted.** It teaches people that your time, your heart, and your health are available on demand, regardless of whether you're okay.

Setting boundaries isn't the painful thing. **Staying boundaryless is.** Every time you choose not to honor your limits, you chip away at the relationship you have with yourself. But every time you set a boundary, no matter how small, you're sending a new message: *I'm here. I* *matter. I'm willing to care for myself first so I can show up stronger, clearer, and more whole for everything else.*

And that? That's not selfish. That's healing.

A Time I Didn't Set a Boundary (and Paid for It)
It's easy to talk about boundaries now with strength and clarity. But it wasn't always like that for me. There was a time, especially early in my healing, when I still believed that saying yes was the safer, kinder thing to do.

Not long after my brain surgery, when my body was still deep in recovery mode, someone asked me for a favor. A small thing, objectively. Just a quick meeting. Just an hour of my time. Just a little emotional energy. At least, that's how they made it sound.

Inside, my body was already screaming no. I was still dealing with migraines, with fatigue that hit like a truck, with brain fog that made simple conversations feel like climbing a mountain, blood sugar dysregulation, and nausea. I knew I needed rest. I knew I wasn't ready.

But somewhere deep inside, that old story started playing. *They need you. Don't let them down.* I told myself, *It's just an hour. You can push through.* So I said yes.

And for that one hour, I smiled, nodded, and gave what I could. On the outside, I looked fine. On the inside, I was white-knuckling it through every second. Even though I put mind over matter in the moment, my body paid the price for the next week.

My energy crashed. My pain levels spiked. The little ground I had clawed back in my recovery slid away under my feet. All because I couldn't bear the idea of disappointing someone, even when it meant abandoning myself.

That was a turning point for me. I realized that the real betrayal wasn't disappointing someone else. It was abandoning my own healing, my own health, my own hard-won progress.

Setting boundaries isn't selfish. It's survival. It's not about being rude. It's about refusing to bleed out emotionally for the comfort of others.

And once you see the cost clearly, you can't unsee it. That was one of the last times I traded my peace for approval. And I am a better, stronger, healthier person for it.

That experience taught me something I'll never forget. Clear, kind communication isn't optional when you're protecting your peace. It's essential. And the good news is, you don't have to guess or stumble through it. You can prepare your words ahead of time, practice them, and use them like anchors when the moment comes.

Scripts for Boundary-Setting: Protecting Without Punishing

Let's walk through what setting healthy, real-world boundaries can actually sound like. Boundaries don't have to sound harsh. You don't have to deliver them with a hammer. You can be clear *and* kind at the same time. Here are some examples.

Family

I love you, and I'm not available for that conversation right now.

That topic doesn't feel helpful for me to discuss. Let's talk about something else.

Friendship

I want to support you, but I need to be honest about what I can realistically give right now.

I care about you, but I'm not able to take on emotional support today. Can we catch up another time?

Work

I'm happy to help with this project. To stay on schedule, I'll need to prioritize after I finish my current assignments.

I can contribute, but I'll need clear expectations and a realistic deadline.

Partnerships

I need some time alone to recharge tonight. It's not about you—it's something I'm giving myself.

I want to have this conversation, but I need a little time to collect my thoughts so I can show up the way I want to.

Notice, no over-apologizing. No over-explaining. No justifying why your boundary is *valid.* Just short, clear, kind statements. That's it. When you communicate your limits with respect for yourself and others, you invite healthier dynamics everywhere you go.

If you find yourself wanting even more support around how to say these things, or you need help finding the exact words for trickier situations, I wrote an entire book on this topic called *Conversational Boundaries.*

It's filled with real-world scripts, examples, and strategies to help you set clear, kind limits without getting tangled up in guilt or confusion. If you're ready to go deeper, I highly recommend grabbing a copy. (You can think of it as your personal training manual for boundary conversations.)

How to Handle Pushback — Without Folding

Here's the uncomfortable truth. **When you start setting boundaries, some people will push back.** Not because you're wrong. But because you're changing a pattern they benefited from.

Pushback doesn't mean the boundary is bad. It means it's working.

Think of it like installing a brand-new fence where there was no fence before. At first, people might lean on it. They might test it. They might grumble about it. That doesn't mean the fence was a bad idea. It means it's doing its job, defining what's yours to protect.

Here's how to handle pushback.

- **Expect it.**
  Discomfort doesn't mean danger. It means growth.

- **Stay calm and consistent.**
  You don't need to match their emotional escalation. Your calm is power.

- **Repeat the boundary without justifying.**
  You're not negotiating your needs. You're communicating them.

- **Detach from needing approval.**
  People's feelings about your boundary are *theirs* to manage, not yours to absorb.

You are not responsible for someone else's discomfort with your growth. You are responsible for protecting the peace you fought to reclaim.

Setting Boundaries Can Feel *Mean* at First

Let's just go ahead and name something most people feel, but few want to admit. **At first, setting boundaries can feel mean.** Even when you're being kind. Even when you're being clear. Even when you're doing everything right.

Because if you spent years (or decades) equating love with self-sacrifice, or peace with silence, or worthiness with overgiving, then speaking up for your needs is going to feel wrong at first. Not because it *is* wrong. Because it's *new*.

Old programming whispers, *You're being selfish.* It pokes the guilt button with, *You're hurting people.* Or how about a little fear and abandonment? *You're going to lose them.*

New truth answers from grounded clarity.

- *You're protecting the connection you're healthy enough to sustain.*

- *You're making love and respect go hand-in-hand, not stand in opposition.*

- *You're showing up for yourself so you can show up for others more fully and freely.*

Feeling guilty doesn't mean you're doing boundaries wrong. It often means you're doing them exactly right. You're not being mean. You're being clear. There's a world of difference. And over time, your nervous system will catch up with your new truth.

Boundaries without clarity confuse people. Boundaries without follow-through train people to ignore you. The key is **consistency**.

I've worked with clients who said things like, *I've told my mom a hundred times not to comment on my body, but she still does!* And when we explored it, we found that the *boundary* was usually just a **plea**, *Please don't say that.* Followed by compliance. Smiling through it. Changing the subject. No consequence.

A boundary that isn't enforced is just a wish. So let's talk about enforcement, because this is where most people panic. Enforcement doesn't mean aggression. It means **action.** If someone continues to violate your boundary after you've clearly expressed it, you follow through with behavior change.

- If a friend keeps canceling last minute, you stop rearranging your schedule for them.

- If a family member keeps making passive-aggressive comments, you cut the conversation short or leave the room.

- If a partner violates your emotional or physical safety, you seek support and step away.

This isn't about punishment. It's about protection. And yes, it might upset people. But anyone who respects you will also respect your boundaries. Those who don't? They were relying on your lack of boundaries to begin with.

That is the heart of becoming unbothered. You stop dancing around dysfunction. You stop explaining your needs to people committed to misunderstanding them. You stop shrinking for comfort and start standing in clarity. And when you do it often enough, boundaries stop being scary. They become second nature, just like locking your front door before bed.

The Difference Between Guilt and Growth

One of the sneakiest things that trips people up when setting boundaries? **Guilt.** Not because you're doing something wrong, but because you're doing something *different.*

Guilt is the emotional residue left behind when you disrupt an old survival pattern. It feels like: *I'm being mean. I'm selfish. I'm abandoning people.* But more often than not, guilt isn't a sign you're bad. It's a sign you're healing.

Here's the reframe.

- **Guilt says,** *This is unfamiliar.*

- **Growth says,** *This is necessary.*

You're not betraying your values by setting boundaries. You're protecting your future. Every time you say no with kindness, every time you honor your needs without crumbling, you are expanding your capacity for healthier connection, healthier leadership, healthier living.

And yes, sometimes it feels heavy at first. That's okay. You're not losing your heart.□
You're finding your strength.

The Boundary Map: Identify, Choose, Follow Through

Setting a boundary doesn't have to be complicated. It's not a magic trick. It's a map. It starts with knowing three things: where you are, where you want to go, and how you're going to get there.

Step 1: Identify the Need
Ask yourself:

- What am I protecting?

- Time? Energy? Peace? Emotional safety?

Get clear on what's truly at stake. Not just what feels urgent in the moment.

Step 2: Choose the Wording

Decide ahead of time how you will communicate.

- Short.

- Clear.

- Kind.

You already practiced some examples earlier. You don't need to over-explain or apologize for needing what you need.

Step 3: Follow Through

This is the part where emotional strength gets built.

- Communicate it once.

- Hold it consistently.

- Detach from others' reactions.

Consistency creates safety. Not just for you, but for everyone around you.

Quick visual tip:

Think of a GPS recalculating when you take a different route. It doesn't scream. It doesn't shame you. It just says, *Rerouting.* And it keeps going.

Your boundaries can work the same way. No need to escalate. No need to collapse. Just *reroute* back to your peace and keep moving forward.

Real-Life Example: Walking the Boundary Map

Let's say you realize you're feeling exhausted every evening because your family expects you to jump into conversations or errands the second you walk in the door after work.

Boundary Map Walk-Through

- **Identify the Need**

  I need quiet, solo time to decompress after work so I don't carry stress into my family interactions.

- **Choose the Wording**

  I'm going to start taking thirty minutes for myself

after I get home, before I'm available for conversation or plans. It helps me show up better for everyone.

- **Follow Through**

  When you walk in the door, you kindly remind them: *I'm taking my thirty minutes. I'll catch up with you after.* If they push back, you gently but firmly repeat: *I'll be available after my thirty minutes.*

No drama. No lectures. Just calm, kind, consistent follow-through. And with time, it becomes normal. Not a battle. Not a guilt trip. Just a healthy boundary that serves everyone better.

Using the Boundary Map over and over rewires your nervous system, your relationships, and your entire life toward peace, clarity, and sustainability. Boundaries stop being hard conversations. They start becoming a normal part of loving yourself *and* others better.

Boundaries Build Healthier Connections

Setting boundaries isn't about cutting people off. It's about choosing yourself first, so you can love others better from a place of wholeness, not depletion. You're not setting boundaries to push people away. You're setting them to create pathways where real connection, respect, and sustainability can exist.

Every time you communicate your needs clearly and kindly, you're not just protecting yourself. You're giving others a chance to meet you in truth. Every boundary, no matter how small, is your inner voice saying, *My energy matters. My time matters. My peace matters. My voice matters.*

Not everyone will celebrate your boundaries. And that's okay. Your life isn't built on other people's approval. It's built on your truth. Some will rise to meet you. Some won't. Either way, you're standing in your worth. And that's a victory every single time.

Remember, you are not just protecting yourself. You're inviting healthier, stronger, more sustainable connections into your life. And that starts with one clear sentence, one quiet act of courage, one boundary at a time.

If setting boundaries feels scary sometimes, that's normal. You're not just changing conversations. You're changing generational patterns, old habits, and survival instincts that once protected you. Be gentle with yourself.

It's okay if your voice shakes. It's okay if your stomach flips. It's okay if you second-guess yourself afterward. The point isn't perfection. The point is persistence.

Every time you honor your energy, your limits, your worth, you teach the world how to love you better. You teach yourself how to love you better. Boundaries aren't walls to keep love out. They're bridges that let healthy love in. **And you are more than worthy of that.**

Every boundary you set is an act of self-respect, not selfishness. You're not pushing people away. You're protecting the peace you fought to build.

Keep building. You're becoming unbothered for a reason.

Try This Toolkit

Journal Prompt

What's one conversation you've been avoiding? What do you fear might happen if you speak your truth?

2-Minute Mindset Reframe

Clear communication isn't rude. It's respectful. Silence might keep things calm, but it often keeps things broken. Your voice deserves to be part of the solution.

Sensory Reset

Breathe in through your nose for four counts, hold for four, exhale through pursed lips for six. As you exhale, release tension from your jaw and shoulders. This calms your nervous system so you can speak, not react.

Power Statement

I can be both kind and clear. I don't have to choose.

Anchoring Truth

Setting boundaries doesn't mean you're being mean, rigid, or unkind. It means you're being honest with yourself and with others. When your yes is authentic and your no is firm, you're not creating conflict. You're creating clarity.

Let your 'Yes' be yes, and your 'No,' no. – **Matthew 5:37**

This ancient wisdom isn't about being polite. It's about being aligned. You don't owe anyone elaborate explanations for choosing your peace. Boundaries spoken with integrity have a power that doesn't need to shout.

Detachment doesn't mean you stop caring. It means you stop trying to control.

—Unknown

CHAPTER 8
STEP FOUR – DETACHMENT STRATEGIES

Picture this. You're in the middle of a conversation, and you feel it, that tightness in your chest, the quickening of your thoughts, the sudden urge to justify or explode. That's your button being pushed.

Now imagine this instead: You smile. You breathe. You disengage. You stay anchored.

That's the art of detachment. Sometimes, the greatest act of strength isn't fighting harder. It's letting go. It's refusing to keep answering every emotional knock like your peace is on the line. It's realizing that other people's chaos is not your emergency.

You can care *without carrying*. You can love someone and still not absorb their chaos. You can be present, but not entangled. Detachment is often misunderstood. People think it means not caring, being cold, or shutting down.

But true detachment is none of those things. Detachment is clarity. Detachment is emotional freedom. Detachment is choosing what *not* to hold.

If boundaries are about where your energy begins and ends, detachment is what keeps you from dragging other people's emotions into your internal space. It says:

- *That's yours. This is mine.*

- *I can support you, but I don't have to solve this for you.*

- *I can witness your pain without drowning in it.*

Detachment is what keeps you from emotionally bleeding out while trying to save people who aren't trying to save themselves. This chapter is about protecting your energy, reclaiming your emotional real estate, and learning the beautiful, liberating art of healthy detachment.

Emotional Detachment vs. Avoidance

Here's the truth you need up front. **Detachment is not avoidance.** Avoidance is rooted in fear. Detachment is rooted in strength. It's not indifference. It's not emotional coldness. It's the decision to stop bleeding energy over things you can't control.

So what does detachment actually look like? It's in the moment you pause instead of jumping in to fix. It's in letting the phone ring when you don't have capacity. It's in reminding yourself: *Their reaction is not my responsibility.*

Detachment says:

I can be present without being pulled under.

Avoidance says:

I'm too overwhelmed, so I'm running away.

Detachment is a conscious emotional boundary. It keeps your nervous system regulated. It preserves your clarity and protects your peace.

Avoidance, by contrast, is emotional shutdown. It buries the discomfort instead of dealing with it.□
And buried emotions don't die quietly—they leak out later as resentment, health issues, or explosive reactions.

Detachment helps you stay awake, compassionate, and anchored. Avoidance cuts you off from your own life force.

When you detach, you honor both yourself and others by staying connected, but not consumed.

When Avoidance Cost Me, and Detachment Saved Me

I'm going to be real and vulnerable in this next part. This is my personal experience as I lived it, and I share it here as part of my own healing journey.

For a long time, I confused avoidance with survival. During the last years of my marriage, a fifteen-year relationship marked by severe emotional, psychological, and physical abuse, I became a master at staying silent. Not peaceful. Not detached. Silent.

At first, it was small things, like choosing not to respond to the jabs, walking away from the gaslighting, biting my tongue to *keep the peace*. It felt like strength at the time. Like wisdom. Like survival.

But over time, the silence grew louder inside me than the abuse happening outside of me. I stopped speaking. Not just carefully, but almost entirely. For the better part of a year, I lived in near-complete emotional silence. Not because I didn't have words. But because I knew that no matter what I said, the outcome would be the same, or worse.

I thought I was protecting myself by avoiding conflict. But in truth, I was slowly disappearing. My body started keeping the score, my voice was too tired to tell. The stress eroded my health. The emotional exhaustion bled into physical symptoms I couldn't ignore anymore.

I didn't recognize it fully at the time, but what I was practicing wasn't healthy detachment. It was dangerous avoidance. And the longer I stayed silent, the more damage I allowed to take root inside me.

Leaving that relationship was the hardest thing I've ever done. But learning to *detach,* to stop internalizing his storms, to stop trying to survive by shrinking, to stop equating silence with safety, *that* was what ultimately saved my life. Healthy detachment taught me that true safety isn't built by disappearing. It's built by protecting your peace even if your voice shakes. It's built by staying present to yourself, even if others refuse to meet you there.

Avoidance cost me years. Detachment gave me my life back. And now, I fight for my peace with the same fierce love I once reserved only for others.

Because no matter who knocks, no matter who pushes, no matter who rages at the door...

I know whose house this is now. And it's mine to protect.

When It Feels Unnatural to Let Go

Here's the part people don't talk about enough. **At first, letting go feels unnatural.** Especially if you grew up learning that love means fixing. That loyalty means staying silent. That worthiness means absorbing everything without complaint.

When you start practicing detachment, it can feel cold. Selfish. Even a little cruel. Not because you're doing it wrong. But because you're doing it *new*.

Your nervous system isn't used to watching a storm rage and staying seated. Your heart isn't used to witnessing someone's disappointment without rushing to fix it. Your mind isn't used to protecting your peace without guilt.

It's not natural yet because it's not familiar yet. Healing often feels wrong at first. Because for so long, dysfunction felt normal. This is where most people get stuck, believing that the discomfort of growth means they're making a mistake.

It's not a mistake. It's a recalibration. Letting go of what's not yours to carry isn't betrayal. It's loyalty to yourself, your healing, and your future. And the more you practice it, the more natural it will feel to stay rooted while the world whirls around you. **You're not becoming harder. You're becoming wiser.**

Protecting Your Energy Without Going Numb

You don't need to numb out or shut down to survive other people's chaos. You don't have to build walls that shut love out.

Healthy detachment is about building **emotional filters**, not emotional bunkers. Imagine your emotional boundaries like a gentle but flexible shield.

- It allows connection.

- It allows care.

- But it doesn't allow trespassing.

You can listen without absorbing. You can care without carrying. You can witness without reacting.

Personal reminder:
I had to learn this lesson the hard way, especially during my recovery season. I realized that if I didn't consciously protect my energy, I was handing it out like free samples at a grocery store, gone before I even realized it.

Protecting your energy isn't selfish. It's sacred. You don't owe anyone unlimited access to your mind, heart, or spirit. No matter how loudly they knock.

Staying Grounded When Others Escalate

When someone else spirals, your nervous system naturally wants to spiral too. (*Hello, mirror neurons.*)

Grounding practices pull you back to yourself.

- **Feel your feet on the ground.**
  Press your toes into your shoes. Feel the floor hold you up.

- **Slow your breathing.**
  One deep exhale sends the message: *I am safe.*

- **Lower your voice.**

Lowering your tone calms your nervous system *and* signals non-threat to the other person.

- **Repeat a grounding phrase mentally.**

- *This is about them, not me.*

- *Their storm is not my emergency.*

- *I can stay rooted, no matter how hard the wind blows.*
  You don't have to match other people's chaos. You can let their storm rage—and still stand dry, calm, and rooted on your own solid ground.

Why Staying Grounded Feels So Hard (Hint: Mirror Neurons)

There's actually a biological reason why staying calm when someone else escalates feels so hard. Your brain has a copy-cat reflex. It's called **mirror neurons**. I mentioned these before, but let's dig deeper into what they are and how they impact you.

Mirror neurons are special brain cells that activate both when you perform an action *and* when you observe someone else performing it. They're part of what makes empathy possible. Your brain naturally *mirrors* the emotional state you see in others.

Which is beautiful when someone's laughing joyfully. Not so great when someone's losing their mind in front of you. When someone's angry, anxious, or escalating, your mirror neurons instinctively want to pull you into the same emotional state, *matching their energy without you even realizing it.*

That's why it can feel like you're getting sucked into their chaos without even choosing it. **But here's the good news.** Once you're aware of this, you can outsmart it.

You can override the mirroring reflex by:

- Grounding your body first (feet flat, shoulders relaxed)

- Slowing your breathing

- Lowering your voice instead of raising it

- Repeating an anchoring phrase like, *Their storm is not my emergency.*

Try the UNHOOK Method if you need a specific strategy to guide you through these moments.

U – **Understand your trigger**

N – **Name the emotional charge**

H – **Hold space for your nervous system**

O – **Observe, don't absorb**

O – **Opt out of the dynamic**

K – **Keep your energy anchored in you**

You don't have to mirror their chaos. You can model calm instead. Your nervous system can become the stronger signal.

Freedom in Letting Go

One of the most powerful things you'll ever learn about peace? You don't have to fix everyone's misunderstanding. You don't have to chase every narrative.

You can allow people:

- To misunderstand you

- To judge you

- To project onto you

- To have their own emotional weather

Letting go of the need to control other people's perceptions is how you reclaim your peace. But, and this is critical, letting go doesn't mean tolerating mistreatment. You are allowed to protect your peace and your dignity at the same time.

You are not a doormat. You are not a dumping ground. You are not required to stay in places where your peace is consistently violated.

Detachment means: *I will not carry your emotions or your stories about me.* It does **not** mean: *I will silently tolerate disrespect, abuse, or mistreatment.* Detachment gives you clarity. It gives you a choice. It gives you the strength to say, *I see what's happening, and I choose myself anyway.*

Care, but don't carry. Love, but don't lose yourself. Detachment isn't about shutting down; it's about showing up without losing yourself.

When you master the art of letting go, you conserve your energy for the places where love, respect, and reciprocity can actually flourish. You are not here to chase misunderstandings or fix everyone's feelings. You are here to protect the peace you fought so hard to reclaim.

Visualization: The Disconnected Doorbell, Revisited

Remember GG's disconnected doorbell? The one you could push all day, all night, by the most frantic visitor, and it didn't matter, because the signal never reached inside? Inside the house, life went on quietly. Peacefully. Unaffected. That's the emotional reality you're building now.

Visualize it. You're inside your inner home. The air is calm. Maybe a soft breeze stirs the curtains. You hear your favorite song playing faintly in the background. Maybe there's the scent of something comforting coming from the kitchen (fresh coffee, cinnamon lingering). You feel grounded and at peace.

Outside, someone is hammering on the doorbell. Banging on the door. Pacing, huffing, fussing. Pushing every button they can find. Maybe even shouting. But you don't react. You barely even register the noise. Because inside, you know, the wiring's been disconnected.

Old you would've rushed to the door, heart pounding, ready to fix, explain, justify. New you? You smile. You don't even flinch when the knocking starts. You know, *not every knock deserves an answer.* You stay rooted inside your peace, and trust that whatever's happening outside doesn't have to disturb your inner world.

You're not being rude. You're not ignoring real emergencies. You're simply no longer making chaos a priority. You sip your coffee. You stretch. You pick up the book you were reading, or return to the conversation you were having with someone who is safe. You stay connected to your life. To your peace. To your purpose. The banging fades into background noise, and eventually, if you stay rooted long enough, it fades out entirely.

That's emotional freedom. And you're getting stronger at living it every day. You didn't have to slam the door. You didn't have to shout through it. You didn't have to perform your pain or your proof. Because when your emotional doorbell is disconnected from other people's panic, you don't live at the mercy of every knock. **You live in freedom.**

Micro-Practice: Emotional Anchoring Phrase

When you feel yourself getting pulled toward the door, when the knock feels too loud, when the urge to explain, defend, or fix starts buzzing under your skin... **Pause.**

Place a hand over your heart or press your feet into the floor. Take one slow breath. And whisper to yourself, *Not everything deserves my energy.* Or maybe, *I can notice without absorbing.* Or, an old favorite of mine, *Their urgency is not my emergency.*

Let the words anchor you back into your body. Back into your breath. Back into your truth. Because the truth is, you don't owe every knock a response. You don't owe every story your spirit.

Sometimes strength looks like staying seated in your peace while the world fumbles for a way in. Practice your anchoring phrase a few times a day. Even when things are calm. That way, when the storm comes, your body already knows the way back home.

Reflection: What Does Peace Feel Like in Your Body?

Peace isn't just a mental concept. It's a physical experience. Tune in. Ask yourself the following questions.

- **Where does peace live in my body?**
  Chest? Shoulders? Hands?

- **How does my breath feel when I'm ground-**

ed?

Slow? Full? Easy?

- **What small practices help me return to peace quickly?**
  A stretch? A hand over my heart? A short prayer or mantra?

Write it down. Describe it like you're giving directions to a friend. Because the more familiar you become with the *felt* experience of peace, the easier it will be to find your way back, even when life gets loud.

Emotional Reframing: Choosing Detachment Is Choosing Love for Yourself

It's easy to think that detachment means giving up. Giving up on the relationship. Giving up on loyalty. Giving up on hope. But that's not what healthy detachment is at all.

Healthy detachment isn't abandoning others. It's refusing to abandon yourself.

It's saying,

- *I will not lose myself trying to hold you together.*

- *I will not sacrifice my peace to soothe your chaos.*

- *I will love myself enough to stay grounded, even when others are ungrounded.*

Choosing detachment is choosing love. Love for your nervous system. Love for your sanity. Love for your future.

It's trusting that other people have the right to their journey, their storms, and their misunderstandings. And you have the right to your clarity, your boundaries, and your peace. You're not giving up on love when you detach. You're giving love its healthiest chance to breathe.

Because real love, love that honors dignity, wholeness, and freedom, can only exist where there is space to choose, not pressure to perform. Every time you choose detachment over reactivity, you're choosing to live from love, not fear. And you're getting stronger at it every single time.

Protect Your Peace Like It's Priceless

Detachment doesn't mean caring less. It means caring smarter. It means refusing to let chaos decide the quality of your day. It means refusing to let old stories steal your present. It means refusing to let other people's noise drown out your truth.

You don't have to slam the door on the world. You just have to stop answering every knock. **You can't control who rings the doorbell. But you can absolutely control whether you answer.**

And every time you choose yourself, you build a stronger, steadier, more unbothered life. Keep choosing peace. You're getting closer every day.

The Shift Has Already Begun

Change doesn't always announce itself with trumpets. Sometimes it's as quiet as a new choice you didn't make before.

You might not even realize it yet, but the shift has already started.

The moment you noticed your buttons instead of automatically reacting, the moment you paused instead of chasing, the moment you chose your peace over your old patterns, you began building something no one can take away from you.

You've done more than survive the noise. You've started disconnecting the doorbell. You're not at the mercy of every knock anymore. You're no longer sprinting to the door, breathless, heart racing, every time someone demands your energy.

You're learning that your life, your energy, your peace, your mind, is sacred ground. And you are the only one who gets to decide what crosses it.

From here on out, it's not about becoming someone brand-new. It's about remembering who you were before the world taught you to flinch, chase, collapse, or explain.

The Unbothered Button isn't something you earn. It's something you build, choice by choice, breath by breath, boundary by boundary. And whether you can feel it yet or not, **you're already becoming unbothered.** Let's keep going.

Small shifts create seismic change over time. You're already moving.

Try This Toolkit

Journal Prompt
Who pushes back the most when you assert your boundaries? What does that reveal about the dynamic you're shifting?

2-Minute Mindset Reframe

Pushback doesn't mean your boundary is wrong. It means it's working. Discomfort is often the first sign of growth, not failure.

Sensory Reset

Lightly press your feet into the floor or ground. Notice the sensation of stability. Remind yourself: *I am supported.* Repeat as needed when you feel shaken or second-guessing your stance.

Power Statement

Their resistance is not my responsibility. My alignment is.

Anchoring Truth

There comes a point in your healing where you realize that not every battle deserves your energy. Detaching doesn't mean you've given up. It means you've handed it over. You're no longer trying to fix, prove, or convince. You're choosing stillness over struggle.

The Lord will fight for you; you need only to be still.
– Exodus 14:14

There is peace in knowing that you don't have to carry it all. Stillness isn't weakness—it's a spiritual strategy. Letting go is sometimes the strongest thing you can do.

PART III

Living Unbothered

You can't stop the waves, but you can learn how to surf. — Jon Kabat-Zinn

CHAPTER 9
CREATING A RESILIENCE TOOLBOX

You've done the inner work. You've identified your buttons. You've started challenging your thoughts. You're setting boundaries and detaching with clarity. But here's the truth... life will still be life.

No one gets through life without storms. The goal was never to build a life so quiet, so controlled, that nothing ever shakes you. The real freedom is knowing that even when the wind picks up, even when the waves rise, you have everything you need to stay standing.

Resilience isn't about becoming untouchable. It's about becoming unshakable. Life isn't about learning how to avoid storms. It's about learning how to stay standing when they hit. Storms will come. Plans will unravel. People will still, occasionally, press your buttons with the force of a toddler smashing an elevator panel.

You can't control that. But you can build something inside yourself that doesn't break every time the winds pick up. **That something is resilience.**

And the good news is, resilience isn't some mystical trait you either have or don't. It's not a birthright. It's not reserved for people who meditate on mountaintops or live minimalist Instagram lives.

Resilience is a skill. It's a toolbox you build, one small practice, one strong decision, one tiny emotional reset at a time. And today, you're going to start filling yours.

- Not with *perfect* routines you'll abandon after three days.

- Not with ten-step regimens that feel like another full-time job.

- **With simple, real, flexible tools that fit into your actual life.**

These are practices you can reach for when you feel yourself slipping back into old patterns. Tools you can trust when you're tired, triggered, or tempted to spiral. Not all of these will fit everyone, but you don't need all of them. What matters is building a personalized set of tools that meet you where you are and remind you who you are. Because you don't need to become a different person to be resilient. You just need a better set of tools.

Defining Emotional Resilience

Before we build your toolbox, let's get clear on what we're actually building. **Emotional resilience isn't about pretending everything's fine.** It's not about slapping on a positive quote and ignoring your reality. It's not about being stoic or superhuman or never feeling triggered again.

Emotional resilience is about feeling disruption and recovering your center faster. It allows you to experience discomfort while remembering it's not dangerous. It's about facing emotional storms and knowing you can survive without losing yourself.

Resilience IS flexibility, not perfection. It's bending without breaking. Recovering without disappearing.

Resilience IS NOT suppressing your emotions. Or forcing yourself to stay silent to *keep the peace.* And definitely not judging yourself every time you feel thrown off.

You're not here to become emotionless. You're here to become *unshakable*, even when emotions show up, as they inevitably will.

Quick Nerd Moment

(You know I can't help myself.) Psychologists have found that emotional resilience isn't just a *nice-to-have* personality trait. It's a **neurological skill** that strengthens specific neural pathways tied to stress recovery, emotional regulation, and even physical health.

In other words, the more you practice resilience, the easier and faster your brain becomes at **calming itself down**, **shifting perspective**, and **resetting emotional balance**, without white-knuckling it. Which means the tools you're about to learn don't just help you survive the next storm. They actually rewire your brain for strength you'll carry for the rest of your life.

Core Self-Care Strategies

Before we start stacking tools into your resilience toolbox, you need a strong foundation to hold it all together. And that foundation is built on something a lot simpler (and less glamorous) than people want to admit. **Self-care.**

Not spa-day, scented-candle, escape-your-life self-care. Real self-care. Daily choices that protect your brain, your body, and your emotional stamina so you can actually handle life without crumbling.

If you've ever felt like you *should* be more resilient but couldn't seem to get there, this is why. You can't build emotional strength if your basic physical and emotional needs are running on empty. Resilience doesn't grow out of thin air. It grows out of how you treat yourself on ordinary Tuesday mornings when nobody's watching.

Let's break it down simply into three parts.

Physical Self-Care: Guarding Your Energy Supply

You can't regulate your emotions if your body is running on fumes. There are **three physical anchors every resilient person protects fiercely.**

- **Sleep**

  - Your brain processes emotional information *while* you sleep.

  - Without enough, emotional regulation goes

out the window.

- ○ Protect your sleep like your peace depends on it—because it does.

- **Movement**

  - ○ You don't have to run marathons or become a gym rat.

  - ○ Move your body enough to process stress hormones physically.

  - ○ Even a brisk walk. A stretch session. Dancing around your kitchen counts.

- **Nutrition Basics**

  - ○ Blood sugar rollercoasters = emotional rollercoasters.

  - ○ Steady, simple eating (proteins, healthy fats, less sugar spikes) gives your brain the fuel it needs to stay calm under pressure.

This isn't about *being perfect*. It's about making small, sustainable choices that give your mind and body a fighting chance when life gets loud.

Emotional Hygiene: Clearing the Daily Build-Up

Just like you brush your teeth every day to prevent decay, you need to **process your emotions regularly** to prevent emotional rot. Skipping emotional hygiene is like letting dirty dishes pile up. Eventually, the sink overflows, and suddenly you're screaming about a fork.

Simple emotional hygiene habits that make a big impact.

- **Name your feelings daily.**
  (*Not just good or bad. Get specific: angry, disappointed, lonely, hopeful.*)

- **Process small stuff when it's small.**
  (*A five-minute journal entry. A vent to a trusted friend. A quiet prayer or meditation.*)

- **Release emotional tension physically.**
  (*A deep sigh. A shoulder roll. A cry if you need it. Your body carries what you don't express.*)

Clearing emotional build-up is resilience maintenance. Not weakness. Not drama. Maintenance.

Boundaries as Self-Care: Protecting the Castle

You can have the best sleep, nutrition, and emotional practices in the world, but if you leave your emotional gates wide open to chaos, you're still going to burn out. Remember what you learned in Part II. **Boundaries aren't about shutting people out.** They're about protecting the environment you need to thrive.

Setting and holding boundaries protects:

- Your time

- Your mental space

- Your physical energy

- Your emotional safety

Boundaries don't make you *mean*. They make you sustainable. Think of boundaries like the walls of a beautiful castle. They're not there because the castle hates the world. They're there because what's inside is *precious* and *worth protecting*. You are that precious thing.

Building Your Toolbox

You've built the foundation. Now it's time to start stocking your resilience toolbox with real, usable tools, things you can reach for the moment you feel yourself getting rattled. **This is where resilience shifts from an idea to a daily, livable reality.**

You don't need thirty-seven techniques memorized or a color-coded coping binder. (Unless you want one. In which case, go ahead and make it cute.) You just need a few powerful tools, you know you can lean on. **Tools that fit your life, your energy, and your needs.** Let's build your starter set.

Journaling Prompts for Emotional Clarity

I can almost feel you eyerolling at this suggestion. I know, I know. Journaling is not for everyone. But I want you to remember, you don't have to write novels to benefit from journaling. Sometimes one good question is enough to reset your whole emotional system.

Here are a few prompts you can pull anytime you feel triggered, overwhelmed, or unsettled.

- **What threw me off today, and why?**
  (*Get curious, not judgmental.*)

- **What brought me back to center?**
  (*Anchor to what actually helps, not just what distracts.*)

- **What thought distortion tried to sneak in, and how did I reframe it?**
  (*Catch the story before it spirals.*)

- **What do I need more of, and less of, tomorrow?**
  (*Reset your energy with intention.*)

Small reflections. Big shifts. There's something magical that happens when you pour your thoughts on paper. Your brain realizes it no longer needs to contain all the information.

Quick Science Fun Fact: Journaling and Your Brain

When you journal, even just a few lines, you're actually giving your brain a much-needed release valve. Here's why.

- Your **prefrontal cortex** (the part of your brain responsible for decision-making, focus, and emotional regulation) gets overwhelmed when it tries to juggle too many unprocessed thoughts and feelings at once.

- Writing things down *physically clears mental clutter.*

  It signals to your brain, *You don't have to keep holding all of this in working memory anymore.*

- This frees up cognitive resources—meaning you have more brainpower left to regulate your emotions, shift your perspective, and stay grounded.

In other words, **journaling isn't just emotional venting.** It's **mental decluttering**. And it leaves more room for clarity, calm, and creative problem-solving.

Affirmations to Rewire Your Mindset

Affirmations aren't magic spells. They're reminders. Like mental sticky notes for your brain when stress tries to rewrite the story.

Choose or create affirmations that *actually* resonate, not ones that make you roll your eyes. Here are a few you can borrow, tweak, or rewrite.

- *I am rooted, not reactive.*

- *My peace is my priority.*

- *Discomfort is not danger.*

- *I bend, but I do not break.*

- *Their chaos is not my invitation.*

Pro Tip

Write your favorite on a sticky note. Put it somewhere you'll see it when you're tired, stressed, or tempted to spiral. Maybe the bathroom mirror. Or maybe the dashboard of your car.

The right words, seen at the right moment, can snap you back to center faster than you think.

Relaxation Techniques: Fast Resets for Real Life

You don't need a silent retreat in the woods to reset your nervous system. I'm not saying retreats are bad or a waste of time. They're just not always practical or feasible. You just need a few quick, portable techniques you can use *anywhere life gets loud.*

Here's your starter set to try.

4-7-8 Breathing

- Inhale for 4 counts.

- Hold for 7 counts.

- Exhale slowly for 8 counts.

- Repeat for two to three cycles.

Why it works: It forces your nervous system to downshift out of fight-or-flight.

Progressive Muscle Relaxation (PMR) Basics

- Tense one muscle group (like your fists) for five seconds.

- Release completely.

- Move to another group (shoulders, jaw, etc.)

Why it works: It teaches your body what true relaxation feels like, not just being *less tense*.

Mindfulness Mini-Practice

- Notice 5 things you can see.

- 4 things you can touch.

- 3 things you can hear.

- 2 things you can smell.

- 1 thing you can taste.

Why it works: It yanks your brain out of anxiety loops and back into the present moment.

Friendly Reminder

You don't have to use all of these at once. Pick **one** that feels doable today. Add another when you're ready. Consistency beats complexity.

Design Your Personal Routine

Here's the truth about resilience routines. You don't need a five-hour morning ritual, seventeen color-coded journals, or a new personality to stay grounded. You just need a few small anchors, tiny habits you can lean on when life gets loud.

This isn't about creating another system you'll abandon the second you have a bad day. It's about designing a **flexible, forgiving framework** that supports you, even when you're tired, overwhelmed, or not at your best. This is your personal resilience map. Not someone else's.

Start simple. Adjust when you need to. Celebrate every tiny choice that helps you come back to yourself.

Build Your Micro-Resilience Routine

You're going to create three small touchpoints across your day.

Morning Anchor

Pick **one small thing** you can do to ground yourself before the world gets noisy. Here are a few examples.

- One-minute breathing exercise

- Set an intention. Ex: *I choose peace today.*

- Read your favorite affirmation.

- Journal one sentence about what you want to feel today.

Question to ask yourself: *What helps me feel rooted before the world starts pulling at me?*

Midday Check-In

Pick **one small habit** that helps you reset halfway through the day. This might look like...

- Quick body scan (where am I holding tension?)

- Step outside for five deep breaths of fresh air.

- Drink a glass of water while repeating your anchoring phrase.

- Stretch, move, shake out stuck energy.

Question to ask yourself: *How can I notice my energy before it drains completely?*

Evening Clearing

Pick **one small ritual** to clear emotional clutter before bed. Try something like...

- Write down one thing you're proud of today (even if it's tiny)

- Journal a *brain dump* to release lingering stress

- Gentle breathing or progressive muscle relaxation

- Speak gratitude out loud, even if it's just *I'm grateful I survived today.* (Because sometimes survival is the goal.)

Question to ask yourself: *How can I close the day instead of carrying it into tomorrow?*

You can even jot these down if you need a reminder. Or, you may need to take these anchors a step further and create reminders to engage with them throughout the day. In my clinical practice, I often advise people to set alarms on their phone that signal it's time to check in and anchor their nervous system. This is especially helpful for people who are overwhelmed, struggling with anxiety, and showing signs of mental burnout.

Remember, you're allowed to change your anchors whenever life changes. The goal isn't to create a prison of habits you have to obey. The goal is to create a soft, supportive structure that keeps you steady through the hard days and builds strength on the good ones.

Real-Life Resilience: When the Dog, the Laptop, and Gravity All Collide

Just to prove that even with all the right tools, life still gets loud and messy sometimes...

This morning, I sat at my grandfather's old oak desk, sunlight streaming in the study, laptop plugged in (because, like many of you, my laptop is old and my battery lasts about seventeen minutes these days). I was ready to work. I had a plan. I had flow. Then someone knocked at the door.

My dog, who is normally quite calm and laid back, lost his mind. He started barking, spinning in circles like a furry hurricane. I jumped up, startled, caught my foot in the laptop cord, sent my chair flying backward, unplugged my computer mid-sentence, and nearly crushed both myself and the dog in the chaos.

All because of a knock I didn't even have to answer. Everything in my nervous system screamed, *Panic!* My mind screamed, *Fix it!* My body took over without my consent. *React!*

And for a second, I did. But then I laughed. A lot!

I caught my breath. I looked around at the chaos and realized, **I'm still okay.** Resilience isn't about having a perfect plan. It's not about controlling every knock at the door. It's about breathing through the chaos, resetting when it unplugs you, and choosing to keep going anyway.

Some days, your peace looks polished. Some days, it's messy and sprawling on the floor next to a barking dog. Either way, you're still building strength. And that counts.

Your Resilience Is Built, Not Born

Resilience isn't a one-time achievement. It's not something you find once and then cross off your list. It's daily armor you build with one choice, one habit, one small act of loyalty to yourself at a time.

You don't wake up unbothered because you had a good day yesterday. You wake up unbothered because you've been quietly, consistently choosing to protect your energy, your peace, and your focus. Even when nobody's clapping for you.

You don't need to be perfect. You don't need a flawless routine. You just need to keep showing up for yourself in the small ways that build strength when nobody's looking.

Every time you pause to breathe instead of react, every time you name your feelings instead of bottling them, every time you honor your boundaries instead of abandoning them... You're building a stronger, steadier, wiser version of you.

And here's the best part. **Resilience compounds.** The more you practice it, the more natural it becomes. You're not fragile. You're not broken. You're not behind. You're building something unstoppable.

And the storms don't get the final say anymore. You do.

Try This Toolkit

Journal Prompt

What's one coping skill that has genuinely helped you through hard times? What tool do you tend to forget about when you're overwhelmed?

2-Minute Mindset Reframe

Resilience doesn't mean never breaking. It means knowing how to rebuild. Even slow progress counts when you're showing up on purpose.

Sensory Reset

Choose one small ritual to start your day: light a candle, stretch your arms overhead, sip warm tea with intention, or play a calming song. Ritual creates rhythm, and rhythm creates stability.

Power Statement

I don't have to be unshakable. I just have to keep returning to myself.

You teach people how to treat you by what you allow, what you stop, and what you reinforce.

— Tony Gaskins

CHAPTER 10
HOW TO HANDLE REPEAT BUTTON-PUSHERS

You've explained yourself. Set the boundary. Stayed calm. And yet, they're back. Same button, same pattern. If you've ever wondered, *'How many times do I have to set this boundary before they stop?'*

Some people aren't confused. They understand your boundary just fine. They heard you the first time. They know what you meant. These are your **repeat button-pushers**. Some people will keep testing you, not because you're wrong, but because your growth threatens their comfort.

They just don't like it. They don't like the new version of you that no longer folds, explains, or plays small to keep the peace. They don't like losing the access, control, or emotional power they once had. They don't like that your *yes* is no longer automatic, and that your *no* now comes with clarity and calm. They just preferred the version of you who made things easier for them.

So what do they do? They test you. Again. And again. And again. And the truth is, every emotionally healing person eventually meets this moment. The question in their mind: *What do I do when someone refuses to respect my limits?*

This chapter is for that part of you that's tired of being polite while someone bulldozes your boundaries with a smile. It's for the part of you that still feels tempted to second-guess yourself every time someone says, *You're being difficult,* or, *You used to be so easygoing.* And it's for the part of you that already knows you're not being dramatic. You're not being rigid. You're protecting your peace.

Habitual pushers might not realize the harm they're causing. They've been doing it so long, it's automatic. These people *can* change, but only if they're willing to grow with you. Intentional pushers, on the other hand, know exactly what they're doing. They thrive on your reaction. They don't want growth; they want control. Let's talk about how to deal with both.

Let's talk about what to do when button-pushers just won't quit and how to stay unbothered even when they keep knocking. Because boundaries aren't about convincing others. They are about protecting the peace you've fought hard to build.

Why Some People Keep Testing You

Here's the hard truth. Some people push your buttons because they've benefited from you being *easily pushed*. If you've always been the fixer, the peacekeeper, the over-explainer, the one who absorbs tension just to make things easier, then the second you stop doing that, it messes with their emotional economy.

They resist because they want the old pattern back. Here are a few reasons they might not give up easily.

Control Issues

People who feel powerless in their own lives often look for control elsewhere. They don't like that you've become harder to manipulate or guilt-trip. They see your boundary as a threat, not because it's aggressive, but because it limits their access.

Habitual Roles and Power Dynamics

If you've always been the *easy one* or the *helper* in the relationship, your boundary challenges their role too. They're not just losing comfort. They're losing the identity they built on your compliance.

Insecurity Masked as Dominance

Some button-pushers act bold, but underneath, they're scared. Your growth reflects their stagnation. Your clarity exposes their chaos. So they push. Not because they're confident, but because they're afraid of becoming irrelevant in your life.

You don't need to psychoanalyze every repeat offender in your life. But understanding *why* they push can help you take it *less personally*. This isn't always about you being *too much*. Sometimes it's about you no longer being *easy to manage*. And that, my friend, is growth.

Handling Strategies by Category

Let's be honest, not all boundary violations are created equal. The guilt trip from your mom hits differently than the passive-aggressive coworker email. The friend who says, *If you loved me, you'd...* hits you somewhere your boss never could. So let's break it down.

The Button-Pusher Types

The Tester

- Pushes once... then again... waiting to see if you will cave.

- Example: A friend who keeps inviting you out even after you said no.

The Guilt-Tripper

- Uses obligation, shame, or loyalty to erode your boundary.

- Says: *After everything I have done for you...*

The Gaslighter

- Denies, minimizes, or spins your boundary into a character flaw.

- Says, *You're so sensitive. It was just a joke.*

The Escalator

- Gets louder or more hostile when boundaries are

enforced.

- Raises their voice, sulks, or makes threats.

Here's an example of how this might look in real life. You tell your sister you're not available to babysit this weekend. She texts three more times. Then says, 'It must be nice to have such a flexible life.' That's not a request. That's manipulation. And it's time to stop engaging like it's not.

The Peacekeeper That Forgot Herself

These patterns often start long before adulthood. For many of us, the pressure to be agreeable, helpful, or low-maintenance didn't come out of nowhere. It was trained into us, sometimes by the very people who claimed to love us most. I know that story well.

There's a reason standing my ground used to feel physically painful. Growing up, I learned early that keeping the peace wasn't just a nice thing to do; it was survival. If I stayed agreeable, flexible, and helpful, things stayed mostly calm. If I said no, asked for something different, or questioned the plan, the whole emotional temperature in the room changed instantly.

So I became really good at reading the room. At softening myself. At carrying everyone else's comfort like it was my responsibility. It took me a long time, and a lot of hard conversations, to realize that what I thought was love was actually emotional enmeshment. That what I thought was kindness was often just fear in nicer packaging.

And when I started setting boundaries as an adult? It rocked the system. Suddenly, family members who never had a problem with me before started calling me *too sensitive, too rigid, too distant.*

But I wasn't distant. I was just no longer available to be the emotional shock absorber. Learning to hold my boundary, calmly, consistently, even when it confused or disappointed people I loved, was one of the hardest skills I've ever built. But it's also one of the reasons I'm still standing today.

Peace built on self-erasure isn't peace—it's emotional debt. And eventually, it always comes due.

That's why family button-pushers can be some of the hardest to handle. They don't just challenge your boundary. They challenge the role you've always played.

Family: Guilt Trips and Boundary Bulldozing

Family is where most of us learned to override our boundaries in the first place. So when you start setting them as an adult, it can feel like you're betraying your upbringing, or becoming *the difficult one.*

Common Moves

- *After all I've done for you...*

- *You used to be so close to the family.*

- *You're being selfish.*

What to Do

- Stick to clear, calm statements. Use the *broken record* technique (we'll get to that soon).

- Resist the urge to explain your boundary fourteen different ways. They *heard* you.

Examples of What to Say

- *I understand that's disappointing. I'm still not able to attend.*

- *That doesn't work for me.*

- *I love you. This is what I need to take care of myself.*

Key Reminder

Guilt is not proof that you've done something wrong. It's often just the emotional discomfort of doing something new and necessary.

Coworkers and Peers: Passive-Aggression and Overstepping

In the workplace, boundary pushers are often less obvious, but just as draining. We spend a lot of time in the workplace, so it is important not to downplay the weight of these interactions.

Common Moves

- *I know you're super busy, but could you just...*

- *I went ahead and looped you in on this project - hope that's okay!*

- Withholding information, subtle undermining, taking credit for your work.

What to Do

- Use clear, professional language; tone matters more than length.

- Don't over-apologize or over-explain.

Examples of What to Say

- *Thanks for thinking of me. I'm at capacity right now, so I won't be able to take that on.*

- *For clarity, I'll need that request in writing.*

- *Let's stay within the scope of what was agreed upon.*

Key Reminder
Boundaries at work are professional, not personal. You're not being rude—you're managing your energy and your role.

Overworked, Overgiving, and Finally Done

These dynamics don't just show up at home. Some of the most persistent boundary pushers wear business casual and CC you on things you never agreed to. I learned that the hard way.

I didn't set out to become *the responsible one* at work. It just... happened. I was the one who stayed late. The one who fixed the projects nobody else wanted. The one who answered the late-night and weekend calls. The one who volunteered because, well, if I didn't, who would?

And for a long time, I told myself it was a good thing. Look how reliable I was. Look how valuable I had made myself.

Until the day someone casually forwarded me a massive project. Something way outside my role. Without even asking, they assumed I'd just take it on.

When I pushed back politely, I got the passive-aggressive response, *Wow. I didn't realize you were getting so territorial.*

It stung. And for a minute, I almost caved, like I had done so many times before. I found myself wanting to apologize. I almost took it on just to *keep the peace.* But then I realized, this wasn't about my professionalism. This was about people getting uncomfortable because I stopped making myself endlessly available.

I had taught them to expect boundary-less access to my time and energy. And now I was teaching them something new, my value isn't measured by how much of myself I sacrifice. It wasn't easy at first. There were some awkward silences. Some shifts in dynamics.

But standing my ground didn't just change how they treated me. **It changed how I treated myself.**

Boundaries at work can feel especially tricky because you're balancing clarity with professionalism. But here's the truth: **your value isn't measured by how much of yourself you give away.** And when you stop over-functioning, the people who benefited from it will almost always push back first.

Friends: Emotional Manipulation Disguised as Loyalty

Friendships are tricky because we often assume love = unlimited access. But real friendship honors boundaries. It doesn't bulldoze them.

Common Moves

- *I guess I know where I stand now.*

- *If you were really my friend, you'd...*

- *It must be nice to have the luxury of boundaries.*

What to Do

- Use direct language without guilt.

- Address the *tone* of the manipulation, not just the words.

Examples of What to Say

- *That felt like a guilt trip. Is there something you need to ask directly?*

- *I care about you, but that comment felt unfair.*

- *My boundary isn't a reflection of how much I love you. It's what helps me show up well when I can.*

Key Reminder

If someone ties your worth to how much you sacrifice for them, that's not friendship. That's performance.

The Art of the Broken Record

Repeat button-pushers thrive on one thing: your emotional reaction. They bait you into long explanations. They wait for cracks in your tone. They listen for hesitation, guilt, or the tiniest wiggle room.

Your job? Become the emotional equivalent of a broken record. Say it. Mean it. Repeat it. Not louder. Not meaner. Just firmer.

Why This Works

When you respond to repeated button-pushing with the same calm phrase, again and again, you teach people that **you don't negotiate your peace.** It's not about being robotic. It's about being steady.

The broken record approach **disarms manipulation** because it gives them nothing to grip onto.
No debate. No loopholes. No new angle. Just the same boundary, calmly reinforced.

How to Use It

Let's say your mother keeps asking why you're not attending a family dinner, even though you've already said no. The conversation might sound like this.

- *You: I won't be able to come this weekend.*

- *Her: But your cousins are flying in! Can't you just rearrange things?*

- *You: I won't be able to come this weekend.*

- *Her: You've changed...*

- *You: I won't be able to come this weekend.*

Notice there are no apologies. There's no long backstory. There's no tone shift. You stay steady. You repeat your boundary like it's your voicemail message.

Eventually, the conversation stops being a negotiation and becomes a mirror. They see they're not going to win. And here's the beautiful part. **When you stop justifying, people stop debating.**

Practice Phrases to Use as Broken Records

- *That doesn't work for me.*

- *I'm not available for that.*

- *My answer is still no.*

- *I've already communicated my decision.*

- *This topic isn't up for discussion.*

Pro Tip: Pick one or two that feel natural in your voice. Practice saying them calmly, out loud. The muscle memory helps.

Escalation Plans: When They Keep Pushing

Some people need to be told once. Others need a structured, step-by-step reminder that your boundary wasn't a *suggestion*. This is where having an **escalation plan** comes in. It's not dramatic. It's not reactive. It's **strategy.**

Think of it like this. You're not fighting harder. You're holding firmer. Let's walk through a three-tier response system you can adapt to nearly any relationship.

Tier 1: Gentle Reminder

Use this approach when someone oversteps casually or forgets a previously stated boundary.
Your tone should be calm, kind, but clear. Here are a few examples of what this sounds like.

- *Just a reminder - I'm not available for that.*

- *I already shared my boundary around this, and I'm holding to it.*

- *No change here. Thanks for respecting it.*

This tier assumes goodwill. It gives them a chance to correct themselves without confrontation.

Tier 2: Firm Boundary Setting

This approach is used when you've already reminded them, and they continue pushing. Your tone here needs to be confident, direct, but not hostile. Here are three examples of what this can sound like.

- *I'm no longer explaining this. My answer stands.*

- *This conversation is crossing a line. I won't continue it.*

- *I've made my position clear. Let's move on.*

At this stage, you stop softening your delivery. No more over-explaining. No more emotional cushioning. This is you protecting your peace like it's priceless. Because it is.

Tier 3: Disengagement or Consequences

This tier should be used when the boundary is repeatedly violated *after* you've been clear. Your tone must be steady and final. No theatrics. This approach should sound like the following.

- *Since you're not respecting my boundary, I'm going to take some space.*

- *I'm ending this conversation now. I'll be available when respect is on the table.*

- *This topic is no longer open. If it comes up again, I'll need to end the call.*

You are not threatening. You are following through. **This is where you close the emotional loop.** You're no longer inviting them to understand. You're protecting your nervous system. You don't owe access to people who abuse access.

Important Reminder

Escalation doesn't mean aggression. It means **reinforcing clarity.** And the more consistent you are, the fewer explanations you need over time. Boundaries repeated are boundaries remembered.

The Repeat Offender Plan

Let's talk about *that person.* You know the one. The person who keeps knocking even though you've already closed the door. The one who always finds a new way to circle back to the boundary you've already set. The one who leaves you questioning yourself more than you ever question them.

This is your invitation to stop bracing for the next interaction and start preparing for it. Not in fear. In clarity.

Take a deep breath, and think of someone in your life who has consistently tested your limits. You don't have to fix the relationship today. You just need to bring it into the light so you can stop being blindsided by it. Ask yourself the following questions.

- **What pattern keeps repeating with this person?**
  Is it guilt-tripping, overstepping, or dismissing your no?

- **What do I typically do in response, and how does that leave me feeling?**
  Do you over-explain, cave in, second-guess, shut down?

- **What boundaries have I communicated or need to communicate more clearly?**
  Have you actually said the thing out loud? Or just hoped they'd get the hint?

- **What's my escalation plan moving forward?**
  What's Tier 1, Tier 2, Tier 3 for this relationship?

- **How will I protect my peace if they still refuse to respect it?**
  What's the emotional exit ramp if they continue

to ignore your boundaries?

This isn't about punishment. It's about protection. You're not planning how to *win*. You're deciding how to **stop losing yourself** in someone else's chaos.

This is you choosing emotional strategy over survival mode. This is you stepping out of the reactive cycle and into your unbothered era. Not every relationship can be saved. But your peace? That can absolutely be protected.

You Can't Control the Knocks - Only the Door

At the end of the day, you will never be able to control who knocks. You can't fix the people who guilt-trip, manipulate, or bulldoze. You can't reprogram the boss who oversteps, the family member who guilts, the friend who tests your loyalty.

But you can control **how many times you open the door.** You can decide when to answer, when to repeat yourself calmly, when to hold firm without apology, and when to walk away without explaining. And that choice, your choice, is where your real power lives.

You don't need everyone to like your boundary for it to be valid. You don't need everyone to understand your no for it to be enough. You are allowed to protect your peace without a courtroom-level defense. You are allowed to choose clarity over chaos. You are allowed to choose yourself.

Because the more you stay rooted, the less tempting it becomes to abandon yourself just to make someone else more comfortable. You're not here to be endlessly available for misunderstanding. You're here to live free. And no matter how many times they knock—◻
You are the one holding the key.

Try This Toolkit

Journal Prompt
What pattern keeps repeating with a certain person in your life? What boundary have you tried, or avoided, setting with them?

2-Minute Mindset Reframe
You don't have to keep proving your worth to people committed to misunderstanding you. Repeating the same defense drains your energy. Choose protection over performance.

Sensory Reset

Step away from the situation and rinse your hands under warm water. As you do, imagine releasing the emotional residue that person leaves behind. Visualize peace returning to your body.

Power Statement

I don't argue with patterns. I disengage and protect my peace.

Peace is not the absence of conflict, but the ability to remain grounded within it.

— Dr. Shiloh Werkmeister

CHAPTER 11
LIVING UNBOTHERED

You weren't born reactive. **You were born whole.**
Then came the messages, the roles, the wounds. You learned to flinch, to defend, to shrink. But who you *are,* that never left. It's time to come home to yourself.

Imagine a life where chaos still circles you, but it no longer lives inside you. The emails still come. The texts still demand. The people still push, pull, question, and spin.

But you? You stay steady. Not because life got easier. Not because the button-pushers disappeared. But because you've done the work to **disconnect the emotional wiring they used to tap into.**

You're not numb. You're not cold. You're **clear.** You have space to think before reacting.
You have energy to create instead of explain. You have peace. Not because everything around you is calm, but because *you* are.

This is the power of becoming unbothered. Not because the world stops knocking...

But because **you no longer open the door just because it's loud.** This isn't about becoming someone new. It's about finally returning to yourself. Living unbothered doesn't mean you're never triggered, hurt, or disappointed. It means those things no longer derail you.

Psychological & Physiological Benefits of Becoming Unbothered

Becoming unbothered isn't just about emotional peace. It changes your **entire system.** Mind. Body. Focus. Relationships.

This is a reclaiming. Reclaiming your identity isn't about becoming someone new. It's about returning to who you were before the world told you otherwise.

Roles We Mistake for Identity

Before we begin rebuilding and redefining identity, let's take a look at some of the common roles we mistake for identity. This isn't an exhaustive list, but I bet you will be able to identify yourself in at least one.

The Fixer

- Believes: *If I don't hold it all together, everything will fall apart.*

- Who they really are = Someone worthy of rest, not rescue missions.

The Strong One

- Believes, *I'm not allowed to break down.*

- Who they really are = Someone allowed to be soft, too.

The People-Pleaser

- Believes: *If they like me, I'll be safe.*

- Who they really are = Someone lovable without performance.

I will openly admit to relating to all of these identities at different times in my life. The important thing to remember here is to hold onto the *Who they really are* pieces for each role. We get to define who we are, and it is okay for that definition to change now and again.

Lower Cortisol, Lower Chaos

Let's start with your body, because it feels it first. When your emotional buttons are constantly being pushed, your brain signals your body to brace for impact, over and over again. That means your **nervous system stays on high alert**, and your cortisol (your main stress hormone) stays elevated. Your body doesn't know you're just responding to a text from your sister or a rude coworker; it reacts like you're being chased by a lion.

This leads to fatigue, headaches, anxiety, brain fog, poor sleep, mood swings, inflammation, and more. And over time, these issues can lead to burnout or chronic illness. When you stop letting every knock at the door throw your system into chaos? **Your body finally gets a break.** You sleep more deeply. You breathe easier. You recover faster. You heal.

Increased Focus, Creativity, and Productivity

When you're emotionally overextended, your brain goes into survival mode. It can't think clearly, solve problems, or imagine new possibilities when it's busy scanning for emotional threats. Your brain is bogged down with stress and hormones, making it unable to function at its best.

But when you're unbothered? You get your bandwidth back. Mental clarity sharpens. Decision-making becomes

easier. Creative ideas return. Tasks that used to feel draining take less energy. You finally have space to build, grow,
and dream again. Being unbothered doesn't make you
passive. It makes you **powerfully present.**

Healthier, More Respectful Relationships

Let's be honest: your button-pushers won't all cheer for
your growth. In fact, most of them will complain about
you changing. Many of them will fall away. But the relationships that survive your boundaries? Those are the ones
worth keeping.

When you live unbothered, you no longer tolerate emotional freeloaders. You attract people who communicate
with clarity and mutual respect. You're no longer afraid of
discomfort. You know how to handle it. You're not performing for connection. You're aligned with people who
get the real you.

This is the foundation for healthier partnerships. This is
where you cultivate stronger friendships. Want to be a
clearer parent? You guessed it. Start here. And if you really
want to go further and get ahead, this is where you devel-
op professional relationships with clean emotional lines.
**Boundaries clear the path for deeper connection. Not
less.**

The Day I Didn't Spiral

There was a time when a certain kind of text message could derail my entire day. You know the kind. Passive-aggressive tone. The guilt trip baked right into the *just checking in*. A subtle suggestion that I've somehow disappointed them, even though I've done nothing wrong.

I used to spiral immediately. Re-reading the message. Questioning what I said or didn't say. Feeling like I had to *fix it* even though I wasn't sure what I'd broken.

And then I'd spend the next few hours drafting the *perfect* response. Polite. Emotionally generous. Over-explaining. Trying to smooth everything out while my heart raced and my stomach flipped. But that was before I did the work of disconnecting the emotional button that said, *It's your job to manage everyone else's disappointment.*

Recently, I got one of those messages again. Same tone. Same guilt laced into the words.□
But this time? My body didn't go into fight-or-flight. I didn't take it on. I took a breath. I read the message once. And then I calmly set my phone down and went back to what I was doing.

No guilt. No spiral. No story. Just peace. That's the difference this work makes. It doesn't mean you stop caring. It means you stop sacrificing your mental health just to manage someone else's discomfort.

That moment might seem small from the outside. Just a text. Just a choice. But for me, it was proof.

Proof that the work I'd been doing wasn't just theory. It was showing up in the most ordinary, emotional moments of my life. And that's the beauty of becoming unbothered. It doesn't always look loud. Sometimes it looks like a pause. A breath. A quiet decision not to hand your energy away.

That's when you know it's real. When peace becomes your default, not your performance. When you no longer feel the need to be in control of how others perceive you. When you can be content letting them handle their own feelings. The knowledge that you have the exact right amount of energy to manage your own thoughts, feelings, and actions. When that feels like enough for you. When you stop giving that precious energy away to people who don't value it.

And the best part? That shift isn't reserved for special people or perfect circumstances. **It's available to anyone willing to do the work.**

Living from a Place of Alignment

Here's the secret about living unbothered. It's not that people stop trying to get a reaction out of you. It's that you're no longer available for the tug-of-war. Because now, your reactions are aligned with your values. Not your wounds.

You don't lash out to prove your worth. You don't people-please to keep the peace. You don't chase closure, approval, or understanding. You choose what's true for you. And let other people sit with their own discomfort if they need to. That's not cruelty. That's clarity.

Peace Over Approval

When you're living from a place of alignment, peace becomes more important than being liked. You stop sacrificing your inner calm to manage someone else's reaction. You realize, not every relationship needs rescuing. Not every misunderstanding needs correcting. Not every invitation requires a response.

You don't lose your empathy. You just stop offering it at your own expense. And the incredible thing? The more you live this way, the more you become someone **you** respect. You stop waiting for others to validate your choices, because your nervous system already knows they're the right ones.

Purpose Over Pleasing

Living unbothered doesn't mean you stop caring. It means you care more about your calling than your comfort. You show up for the work you're here to do, whether that's raising kids, running a business, healing your body, or just choosing peace over survival mode.

You stop asking, *What will they think?* And start asking, *What would alignment look like here?* That's how you reclaim your time, your energy, and your clarity.

You stop spiraling over who misunderstood you. You start moving toward what actually matters.

Holding My Seat at the Table I Built

Not long ago, I was sitting in a professional meeting when the energy shifted. You could feel it. The shift from collaborative to competitive, the way a room changes when someone decides you've had *too much* success and they need to bring you back down to size.

A colleague, someone who had always been pleasant enough on the surface, leaned in with a tone that dripped with casual sabotage. *It's interesting how quickly some people are handed opportunities these days.* No eye contact. No names. Just the kind of comment that lands like a disguised accusation. *You didn't earn this. You don't belong here. You got lucky.*

Ten years ago, that would've wrecked me. I would've spent the rest of the day replaying the comment, wondering if I had misunderstood or if everyone else in the room agreed. I would've mentally re-justified my success to myself, every credential, every late night, every piece of work I'd quietly overdelivered on. I would've let someone else's insecurity dictate my worth.

But not this time. Because the truth is, I had earned every bit of that opportunity. I'd worked for it. I'd sacrificed for it. And I reminded myself of that truth in real time. **I didn't let my feelings rewrite the facts.**

What she was trying to diminish wasn't luck. It was the result of hard work she didn't want to do herself. She wanted to be seen as equal, but not at the cost of effort. So instead of rising, she tried to shrink the room.

And I didn't let her. I didn't bite. I didn't explain. I didn't soften or try to make her more comfortable. I held my posture. I clarified what needed to be clarified. And I moved on, calm, clear, and absolutely unbothered.

Because when you live aligned with your truth, you stop negotiating it with people who haven't earned their place beside you.

The Shift: Old You vs. New You

The difference isn't just in what you say now. It's in what you no longer *feel the need* to say. Let me give some examples. See if these resonate with you.

Old me would've over-explained. Typed out the perfect paragraph. Softened the truth to make it easier for someone else to digest. Apologized for taking up space. *Even when I wasn't wrong.*

New me chooses silence when silence is stronger. New me knows that clarity doesn't require explanation. **New me respects her own peace more than she fears being misunderstood.**

Old me needed closure. New me knows that peace is internal. That peace is not something I have to earn by fixing everyone else's discomfort.

I'm not perfect. I still feel the flicker of doubt sometimes. The urge to prove myself, defend my boundary, win them over. But now I have the tools to pause. To breathe. To choose alignment over urgency. That's not just growth. That's emotional evolution.

Maybe you're not all the way there yet, but you're further than you were. If you've ever paused before reacting... If you've said no without a three-paragraph explanation... If you've walked away from guilt and toward peace... That's the work. That's unbothered. And you should be so very proud of yourself. I know I am.

See How Far You've Come

Pause here. Take a breath. And let yourself acknowledge the growth.

You may not be where you want to be yet, but you're no longer where you started. You've been showing up, holding boundaries, breaking patterns, and choosing peace. Even when it felt unfamiliar or uncomfortable.

Ask yourself:

- When was the last time I held my boundary instead of shrinking to make someone else more comfortable?

- What reaction used to wreck me... that no longer holds that power?

- Where in my life have I made space for calm on purpose?

- What does being unbothered look like for me today, in real life?

This is your moment to celebrate. It is not about perfection, but progress. Because the more you name it, the more it sticks. And the more it sticks, the more naturally it becomes your default setting.

Peace Doesn't Need to Be Loud

I once had a friend who was my emotional opposite. She was bubbly, high-energy, extroverted. Always the life of the party, always texting, always needing connection to feel grounded.

I, on the other hand, am deeply introverted. I recharge in silence. I need space and solitude to think clearly, process emotions, and stay aligned. It's not personal. It's how I'm wired.

But over time, my friend began to take that difference... personally.

When I didn't respond to texts fast enough? I was being distant. When I declined plans to rest instead of going out? I was being selfish. When I asked for space? I was shutting her out.

No matter how kindly I tried to explain my needs, it never seemed to land. She could only interpret the world through *her* lens. *If I needed that much space, it would mean I didn't care. So it must mean that when you need space, you don't care either.* At one point, she even said, *I just feel like I'm always the one reaching out. It's like you don't even try.*

And that's when something shifted in me. Because I *had* been trying. I'd been trying to meet her where she was while still honoring who I was. I'd been trying to show up authentically without abandoning myself. But I realized that no matter how much I bent, it would never be *enough* for someone who only valued love when it looked like *their* version of giving.

So I stopped trying to perform. I stopped over-explaining. I stopped apologizing for not being loud enough, chatty enough, available enough.

And instead, I got honest. I told her I cared deeply, but I wouldn't keep compromising my nervous system to match her rhythm. I would still show up, but I wouldn't show up *differently* just to make her feel more comfortable.

She didn't like it. And truthfully? That friendship faded. But what stayed? My peace. My alignment. My energy. Because when you stop asking others for permission to be who you are, you start attracting relationships that don't need the performance to feel loved.

You Were Never Meant to Fit a Mold

Let this be your reminder. You are not one-size-fits-all. You were never meant to be. Your energy, your pace, your rhythm, your way of relating to the world—it was *intentionally designed*. God didn't make a mistake when He made you quieter than others. He didn't miss the mark when He made you need solitude to feel whole. He didn't forget to install something when you didn't turn out as *on-demand* as others expected you to be. You were crafted with purpose.

And when you honor that, when you stop contorting yourself into what other people need you to be, you start to feel the kind of peace that no approval can buy. **Being unbothered isn't about becoming cold. It's about becoming honest.**

And that honesty? That's what makes space for deeper connection. Because it's not based on performance. It's based on truth.

So if someone doesn't like the version of you that's rooted, whole, and clear... It's okay to let them go. You were never meant to carry everyone's expectations. You were meant to carry peace.

Living Unbothered Isn't Cold - It's Clarity

Let's be clear. Being unbothered doesn't mean you stopped caring—it means you stopped giving your peace to those who didn't know how to hold it.

It doesn't mean you became hard. It means you became steady. **You didn't lose your empathy. You just stopped**

bleeding for people who refused to stop cutting. You didn't shut down. You just stopped letting chaos lead.

You now live from a place of **alignment**. Where your no means no. Where your yes is wholehearted. Where your peace isn't a performance. And your worth isn't up for discussion.

You stopped making your nervous system a landing strip for other people's drama. You stopped giving your energy away like it was free. And in return? You gained focus. You gained clarity. You gained trust in yourself, your voice, and your instincts.

This is what freedom feels like. This is what emotional maturity *looks* like. This is what you've been building with every boundary, every breath, every pause.

You're not *too much*. You're not *too quiet*. You're not *too sensitive*. You are **just enough.** And now? You are free to live like it.

Living unbothered isn't a one-time fix. It's a rhythm. A re-calibration. A way of being that you keep choosing, again and again. You won't always get it right. You'll fall back into old patterns. You'll catch yourself reacting before you realize it.

But now, you have tools. You have awareness. You have a map back home. That's the shift. That's the freedom. You start making choices that feel like alignment, not obligation. You stop performing for people who never had your peace in mind. You stop over-explaining to those who benefit from your confusion. You take up space. Not because you're trying to prove anything, but because it's *yours*.

The Unbothered version of you isn't hardened. It's *healed*. It doesn't armor up—it exudes calm. It's not louder, but *clearer*. It doesn't need revenge. It has *discernment*. It knows that power lies not in controlling others but in protecting your own energy.

Living unbothered isn't just a mindset, it's a lifestyle. And it will change how you show up in every room you enter. Your relationships shift. Your career feels different. Your health improves. Your presence becomes magnetic, not because you're perfect, but because you're centered.

This is your invitation to keep going. To keep choosing calm over chaos. Peace over performance. Purpose over pressure. To trust that when your buttons are disconnected, your soul gets louder. And when your soul is leading, your life becomes *yours* again.

Try This Toolkit

Journal Prompt

What has become easier, lighter, or more peaceful since you began honoring your boundaries? What are you most proud of shifting?

2-Minute Mindset Reframe

Being unbothered isn't apathy, it's clarity. When your worth is no longer up for debate, peace becomes your default, not your reward.

Sensory Reset

Sit still with one hand over your heart and the other on your lower belly. Breathe deeply. With each inhale, say silently, *I am safe.* With each exhale, *I am free.* Let your body memorize this state of ease.

Power Statement

Peace is not something I chase. It's something I choose.

Anchoring Truth

Being unbothered isn't about being cold. It's about being *clear.* It's about holding onto your peace so fiercely that chaos no longer gets a seat at your table. When your mind is anchored, your heart stays steady.

You will keep in perfect peace those whose minds are steadfast, because they trust in you. – **Isaiah 26:3**

Peace isn't passive. It's a byproduct of trust, clarity, and inner alignment. The more you practice choosing what's yours to carry and what's not, the more unshakable your peace becomes.

CHAPTER 12
EXPANDED TOOLS FOR EMPATHS & HSPS

Living Unbothered When You Feel Everything

If you've ever been told *you're too sensitive.* If you've felt like your emotions take up more space than you're allowed. If crowded rooms drain you, certain people overwhelm you, or conflict makes you want to disappear. This chapter is for you.

Some of us are wired to feel more. And that wiring isn't a flaw. It's an intuitive gift. But when left unmanaged, it can become emotional overload.

Let's get something straight. Feeling deeply is not a weakness. In fact, it's often the superpower behind some of the most resilient people you'll ever meet. But if you're an empath or a highly sensitive person (HSP), you've probably been taught to dim that light, manage others' emotions before your own, and sacrifice peace for the sake of keeping the peace.

No more. This chapter is your invitation to reclaim your energy, rewire your guilt, and reset the emotional boundaries that keep you from becoming the version of yourself who can truly live unbothered.

Who Are Empaths and HSPs, Really?

Before we dive into the tools, let's ground this in science, because there's a lot of misinformation floating around about empaths and sensitivity.

An **Empath** absorbs the emotions and energy of others, often without realizing it. Empaths experience a high degree of emotional empathy, which is simply the ability to *feel* the emotions of others, not just understand them cognitively. This is thought to be linked to increased activity in mirror neuron systems, which help us simulate others' experiences in our own brains.

This increased neuron activity comes with both positive and negative consequences. Let's look deeper at how this impacts empaths.

- **The Good**

- Deep connection and compassion

- Powerful intuition

- Ability to sense needs and unspoken pain

- **The Struggle**

  - Prone to emotional exhaustion and burnout

  - Often take on others' emotions as their own

  - Can feel overwhelmed in crowds or high-conflict environments

Empathy is essential to human connection, but **unfiltered empathy** without boundaries can be harmful, especially for those who tend toward people-pleasing, codependency, or hyper-vigilance. **Think of empathy like Wi-Fi. If you don't set a password, everyone drains your bandwidth.**

Now let's talk about HSPs. Coined by psychologist Dr. Elaine Aron, HSPs are people with a **biologically based trait** known as Sensory Processing Sensitivity (SPS). This isn't a diagnosis. It's a **neurological difference** observed in about fifteen to twenty percent of the population.

HSPs have a heightened nervous system response to stimuli (emotionally, physically, environmentally). HSPs process sensory input more deeply, including light, sound, emotions, and even subtleties others miss. Like empaths, HSPs experience both positive and negative ramifications due to the neurological difference in their brain development.

- **The Good**

  - Heightened creativity and insight

  - Deeper appreciation for beauty and meaning

  - Natural emotional intelligence

- **The Struggle**

  - Easily overstimulated or overwhelmed

  - Tendency to ruminate and overthink

  - More sensitive to criticism, conflict, and chaos

For HSPs, sensitivity isn't overreacting; it's high-resolution data processing. But without filters, the constant input can lead to emotional short-circuiting.

Self-Check: Am I an Empath or HSP?

You don't need a clinical label to validate your experience, but self-awareness helps you choose the right tools. Use the statements below to reflect honestly. These aren't diagnostic, but they can help you determine if the content in this chapter applies deeply to you. You can be one or both. And if you're reading this book, chances are high that your sensitivity has shaped your entire life.

Empath Self-Assessment

Check all that apply:

☐ I feel other people's emotions as if they're my own, even when they don't say anything.

☐ I often need alone time after socializing, even if I enjoyed it.

☐ I sometimes feel physically drained by emotional conversations.

☐ People tend to open up to me quickly, even strangers.

☐ I find it hard to watch violent or distressing media.

☐ I've been called *too sensitive* or *too emotional.*

☐ I can sense when something is *off* in a room, even if no one says it out loud.

☐ I have trouble separating my feelings from other people's experiences.

☐ I tend to attract people who need help or healing.

Scoring:

- 0–2: You may not be an empath, but could still have strong emotional intelligence.

- 3–5: You likely have empathic tendencies and may benefit from energetic boundaries.

- 6+: You're likely a full-spectrum empath and should prioritize regular emotional resets and protection tools.

Highly Sensitive Person (HSP) Self-Assessment (Adapted from Dr. Elaine Aron's research.)

Check all that apply:

☐ I am easily overwhelmed by strong sensory input (bright lights, loud noises, chaos).

☐ I am deeply moved by music, art, or beauty in nature.

☐ I notice subtleties in my environment that others miss.

☐ I get rattled when I have a lot to do in a short amount of time.

☐ I avoid violent TV shows or news because they deeply affect me.

☐ I need quiet or alone time to recharge.

☐ I process things deeply and sometimes take longer to make decisions.

☐ I become stressed or anxious when people are watching me.

☐ I get highly affected by caffeine, medications, or pain.

Scoring:

- 0–2: You may have some sensitivity, but not at a heightened level.

- 3–5: You likely have mild to moderate sensitivity and could benefit from lifestyle tweaks.

- 6+: You strongly identify as an HSP and may thrive with sensory regulation and deeper self-care practices.

Now that you have identified whether you likely fit the category of empath or HSP, let's see how this changes the game for you. The truth is, becoming unbothered is different for empaths and Highly Sensitive People (HSPs). It is still doable, but it requires committed focus and dedication.

In a world that praises thick skin, sensitivity can feel like a liability. But here's the truth. **Your sensitivity is not the problem.** It's the lack of tools that's making you feel unsafe. I want to give you some tools. Tools that protect your nervous system, honor your empathy, and help you stay *unbothered,* without shutting down your capacity to feel.

Energetic Boundaries vs. Physical Boundaries

When we think of boundaries, most people imagine the obvious ones: locking your door, saying *no,* avoiding toxic people. These are **physical boundaries**. They protect your body, your space, and your time.

But what about the kind of exhaustion you feel after a group text, or the way you replay someone else's pain for hours after they've left the room? That's an energetic boundary breach. **Energetic boundaries** are the invisible lines between your inner world and everyone else's noise. And for empaths and HSPs, they're non-negotiable.

Try This

- **Visual Shielding:** Imagine a light or bubble surrounding you that only lets in what is loving, kind, and helpful, and filters out the rest.

- **Mantra Reset:** Whisper to yourself, *I can witness without absorbing.*

- **Cord Cutting Practice:** After interactions, mentally (or physically) swipe across your body and say, *I release what isn't mine.*

The more you ground in these practices, the easier it becomes to feel without fusing.

How to Protect Your Peace Without Guilt

Raise your hand if you've ever kept talking to someone who drains you because you felt bad saying no. Yeah, same. Here's the thing: **protecting your peace isn't mean. It's mature.** Peace is not passive, and it doesn't require permission. It's the reward of a person who has done the work to decide what they will and won't allow in their life. You don't owe anyone your burnout, your overstimulation, or your hyper-availability.

Try This

- **Mute button magic:** You don't have to block people to take a break. Mute them. Let your nervous system breathe.

- **Decline-with-love script:** *I care about you, and I'm not in a place to take this on right now.*

- **Create buffer space:** Don't go back-to-back with people or events that demand emotional energy. Schedule recovery like it's sacred, because it is.

Remember: No is a complete sentence, and rest is a revolutionary act for the over-givers.

The Mirror Rule: What's Mine vs. What's Theirs

Empaths often walk into a room and start feeling things they can't explain. It's not always theirs, but they carry it anyway. Here's the rule: *If it didn't start in you, it's not yours to carry.* This is the **Mirror Rule.** Think of it as a mental reframe that helps you sort your emotional inbox before taking action.

Mirror Check Questions

- *Did this originate in me?*

- *Am I trying to fix something I didn't break?*

- *Is their discomfort mine to soothe?*

People will project their pain onto you. Your job is not to become their emotional landfill. Instead, become a mirror. Reflect what's true. Don't absorb what's false.

Try This

- **Ground:** Place your hand over your chest or stomach and name what *you* are feeling.

- **Reflect:** Ask, *Is this mine, or am I matching someone else's energy?*

- **Release:** Inhale. Exhale. *I send this back with love, but it's not mine to hold.*

Final Reminder

Being unbothered as an empath doesn't mean turning off your sensitivity. It means learning how to channel it wisely, intentionally, and without guilt. You are not here to carry the weight of the world. Even though you sometimes feel that way. You are here to shine and protect the light that makes you who *you are.*

Extra toolbox tricks for Empaths and HSPs

TOOL #1: Daily Energy Clearing

Just like you shower your body, you need to clear your emotional energy.□
Here's a quick nighttime ritual:

- Stand or sit in stillness. Close your eyes.

- Imagine a gentle light pouring down over you, dissolving anything you picked up that doesn't belong to you.

- Say (aloud or in your mind): *I release anything that isn't mine.*

This simple ritual helps you reset your energy field and sleep lighter.

TOOL #2: Body-to-Body Boundaries

Empaths often struggle with physical proximity. We can sense shifts in tone, mood, or even posture.

Practice creating physical space when needed:

- Sit across, not beside, someone who drains you.

- Drive your own car to events.

- Avoid hugging or touching when your energy is low.

You don't have to apologize for needing space to stay regulated.

TOOL #3: Media Boundaries

Sensitive people are deeply affected by what they consume. That documentary, that news headline, that story online - it stays with you.

Protect your nervous system:

- Avoid scrolling during emotional vulnerability.

- Curate your feed with intention.

- Watch content that inspires, not drains.

You are not *out of touch* for guarding your peace. You're being responsible.

TOOL #4: Cognitive Anchors for Empaths

When you start absorbing someone else's emotional state, ask yourself:

- Is this mine or theirs?

- Was I feeling this way before they entered the room?

- What do I need to feel safe right now?

These questions create separation between your inner world and their emotional noise. They help you root into yourself.

TOOL #5: Morning Protection Practice

Start your day with intention:

- Visualize a protective bubble or shield around your body.

- Affirm: *I can witness emotion without absorbing it. I can feel without flooding.*

This isn't about blocking love. It's about filtering chaos.

TOOL #6: Choose Gentle Environments

Your nervous system matters. Empaths and HSPs do best with:

- Soft lighting

- Natural surroundings

- Quiet rest spaces

- Gentle textures and sounds

Whenever possible, choose environments that feel like an exhale.

TOOL #7: Compassion Without Codependency

Just because you *can* sense someone's pain doesn't mean it's your job to fix it.
You can be loving without rescuing. You can be kind without contorting.

Try this mantra when you feel yourself overextending:

- *Their healing is their journey. I send love, and I let go.*

Being unbothered doesn't mean you stop feeling. It means you stop carrying what was never yours to

hold. When you learn to manage your sensitivity with intention, you become one of the most grounded, compassionate forces in the room. You are not too much. You are deeply tuned in. And now, you're learning how to stay connected *without collapsing.*

CHAPTER 13
THE B.U.T.T.O.N FRAMEWORK™

I used to think becoming unbothered meant I'd stop getting triggered altogether. But what I've learned, and what I want to offer you here, is that peace doesn't mean you don't react. It means you know how to come back to yourself faster.

I wish I could tell you that I never get triggered anymore. That doing all this healing work means I walk around like some enlightened monk who's completely immune to other people's nonsense. But that wouldn't be honest.

Just a few weeks ago, someone sent me a message that, on the surface, seemed polite. But my body reacted instantly. It wasn't what he said. It was how he said it. That tone. That subtle dismissal. The passive-aggressive phrasing he's mastered like a second language. It was like my nervous system clocked it before my brain could even process it.

For a moment, I was back in the pattern. Heart racing, chest tight, jaw clenching. That familiar loop of: *Maybe I should explain myself again... Maybe I'm overreacting... Why does this still bother me?*...started playing on repeat.

But here's the difference now. I recognized it. And I knew exactly what to do with it.

I walked myself through the B.U.T.T.O.N. Framework, step by step, not perfectly, but intentionally.

I named the button: *feeling dismissed.* I remembered the wiring: *years of gaslighting made me question my own gut.* I tracked the trigger: *heat rising in my face, urge to over-explain.* I rewrote the story: *I don't have to chase understanding to deserve respect.* I reset the boundary: *no need to respond right now.* I grounded myself: *three deep breaths, a hand on my chest, and peppermint oil on my wrists.*

And you know what? What would've taken me out for *days,* mentally replaying the conversation, beating myself up, questioning everything, passed in *hours.* Some days, it passes in minutes. That's what this work does. **It doesn't make you unshakeable because nothing touches you. It makes you unshakeable because you no longer abandon yourself when something does.** Now, I want to teach you how to do the same.

This book began with a broken doorbell. A button that didn't work. A symbol of what it means to be unbothered, someone can press and press, but *you don't react*. Throughout this journey, you've explored awareness, boundaries, detachment, nervous system tools, mindset rewiring, and emotional sovereignty.

But for those who like a clear process, something memorable to anchor into, I created the **B.U.T.T.O.N. Framework**.

Let's be real

Some people know *exactly* what to say to push your buttons. Others do it unintentionally, yet still manage to hijack your energy. And sometimes? You're the one leaning into old programming, pressing your *own* buttons without realizing it.

By now, you've learned the psychology of buttons, identified repeat offenders, and practiced setting boundaries that protect your peace. But transformation doesn't happen in theory. It happens in the *application*. Here's how to make it practical.

This chapter is your personal **Button Audit**. It's where everything you've learned so far gets translated into a step-by-step framework you can use whenever you feel triggered, overwhelmed, or off-center. It's also a framework you'll return to again and again, because the process of becoming unbothered isn't one big moment. It's a series of small, intentional choices that compound over time.

The B.U.T.T.O.N. Framework™

A Six-Step Process to Reclaim Your Emotional Power

B - Button Identified

- *What sets you off?*

Before you can detach from a reaction, you need to name it. Get specific. Is your button around rejection? Criticism? Not feeling heard? Betrayal? Being micromanaged?

Try This:
List three things that consistently provoke a strong emotional reaction in you.

-

-

-

Now pick the one that shows up most often in your re-lationships or daily life. That's your primary button (for now).

U – Understand the Wiring

- *Where did this come from?*

Every button has a backstory. Maybe you were raised to never question authority. Maybe your people-pleasing be-gan as a way to survive emotional chaos. Identifying the source is how we bring compassion into the conversation.

Try This:
Ask yourself,

- When did I first feel this type of hurt?

- Who taught me this was dangerous?

- What was I trying to earn or avoid?

Jot your answers below. No judgment. Just curiosity.

T – Track the Trigger

- *What's happening in your body and brain?*

Your body is often the first to know when a button is getting pressed. Do you get a tight chest? Shaky hands? Go numb? Lash out? Shut down? All of it holds clues.

Try This:

Think of a recent moment when your button was pushed. What were your physical and emotional reactions?

- My body felt:

_____

- I reacted by:

_____

- I said or did:

_____

Understanding your pattern gives you choice.

T – Tell a New Truth

- *What belief keeps this button active and what's the upgrade?*

There's always a story beneath the sting. It might sound like: *I must not be good enough,* or: *If I say no, they'll leave.* Those stories were once protective. Now, they're outdated.

Try This:

- Old belief:

_____

- New truth:

_____

- Affirmation to practice:

_____

Example:

- *Old belief: I have to earn love by being easygoing.*

- *New truth: My needs matter too.*

- *Affirmation: I am allowed to take up space.*

O – Own Your Boundary

- *What do you need in order to stay grounded next*

time?

A disconnected button doesn't mean you stop caring. It means you stop *abandoning yourself* in the process.

Try This:
What boundary supports your new truth?

- Energetic (protect your peace)

- Verbal (speak your needs)

- Physical (leave the room, block the number)☐

- Digital (mute, unfollow, turn off notifications)☐

Write the exact boundary you're going to hold:

N – Neutralize the Button

- *How do you reset and protect your peace going forward?*

This is your grounding plan. Your nervous system needs consistency to believe you're safe.

Try This:
Choose two to three go-to tools to anchor yourself when that button gets tested again:

☐ Breathe slowly for sixty seconds

☐ Shake it off or stretch your body

☐ Journal your triggered thoughts

☐ Use calming essential oils

☐ Go outside barefoot

☐ Speak your affirmation out loud

☐ Phone a grounded friend

☐ Visualize the button disconnecting

You don't need to be perfect. You need to be *present*.
That's what makes you powerful. This isn't a quick fix. It's a daily practice. But if you walk through these six steps, again and again, you will notice a dramatic shift in how you feel, how you respond, and how you protect your peace.

The Final Step: Revisit Often

You're never done with this process, and that's a good thing. The more often you use this audit, the faster you'll rewire your reactions and reclaim your peace. The people who used to control your energy? They'll start to notice something different.

You're not cold. You're not detached. You're just... unbothered.

Want a printable version of this audit?

Download your free Button Audit worksheet at: **www.d rshilohspeaks.com/buttonaudit**

Let's Finish this Together

You're no longer the person who reacts on autopilot. You're someone who notices, reflects, and responds with intention. This framework isn't just a tool. It's a declaration that your peace is no longer up for grabs.

You might still get triggered. You might still feel the sting of an old wound when someone touches it. That doesn't mean you're broken or behind. It means you're *human*.

But with this framework, you now have a way through. A way to honor your nervous system instead of overriding it. A way to protect your peace without performing for it. A way to process what used to spiral, in hours, or even minutes, and move forward without losing yourself.

This is what becoming unbothered looks like in real life. Not perfection. Not avoidance. Just presence. Just peace. Just power.

CHAPTER 14
YOU DID THE WORK.
KEEP DOING IT.

Take a moment. Let it sink in. You didn't just read a book. You walked through fire with grace. You looked at patterns you've lived with for years, maybe your whole life, and said, *No more.*

You learned where your buttons came from. You named them. You took back control of your emotional landscape. You didn't flinch when the truth got uncomfortable.

And most importantly? **You stopped waiting for others to change in order for you to feel peace.** That's not light work. That's *soul* work.

That matters. Because most people don't do this work. They stay reactive. They stay bitter. They stay attached to their buttons because it gives them someone to blame.

But you? You chose the harder path. The more honest path. The path that leads to freedom. And I need you to hear this. **You are allowed to be proud of who you're becoming.**

You're allowed to feel peace. You're allowed to no longer react. You're allowed to walk away from people who expect you to stay broken so they can feel comfortable. This is your permission slip to stop explaining, stop apologizing, and start living like your energy matters, because it does.

This Is the Beginning, Not the End

Becoming unbothered isn't a one-time decision. It's a daily practice. A mindset. A nervous system reset. A quiet act of self-respect that repeats itself over and over, sometimes without applause, often without permission.

Healing isn't linear. You'll slip into old patterns sometimes—and that's okay. Days when the button gets pushed and you feel yourself tense. Days when silence feels uncomfortable, and boundaries feel like conflict. That doesn't mean you failed. That means you're human. This journey is ongoing, and so is your growth.

Just like a muscle, your peace gets stronger the more you protect it. Your clarity gets sharper the more you use it. Your nervous system learns over time: *We're safe now. We're grounded now. We're not going back.*

You Are the Evidence

You may not realize it, but the version of you reading this final chapter? You're different from the one who opened this book. You're more aware. More anchored. More equipped.

You don't chase chaos. You don't justify your needs. You don't hand your peace to the loudest person in the room. You're grounded. You're discerning. You're *unbothered*, not because life is easy, but because you're finally living it on your own terms.

The work you've done isn't invisible. It's in the way you respond instead of react. The way you hold your ground with grace. The way you feel your body exhale after setting a boundary that once would've sent you spiraling.

You are the evidence that emotional freedom is possible. You are the proof that peace doesn't require perfection, just consistency. You are becoming someone your past self didn't know was possible. And I am so, so proud of you.

Carry This With You

When you feel triggered again, because you will, pause. Breathe. Ask yourself, *What's mine, and what's not? What*

*does alignment look like right now? What would my un-
bothered self choose?*

You already know what to do. You've done it again and
again. Now it's about keeping that doorbell unplugged.
Not because people stop knocking, but because you finally
know how to protect your peace.

You Don't Have to Do This Alone

Becoming unbothered doesn't mean becoming isolated.
It doesn't mean walking through life in silence, carrying
everything alone. It means learning how to be grounded *and* supported at the same time. Because even the
strongest among us still need people. We were never meant
to heal in isolation.

*Two are better than one, because they have a good return for
their labor:*
If either of them falls down, one can help the other up.
— Ecclesiastes 4:9–10 (NIV)

God created us for connection. For truth-telling relationships. For emotional safety. For community that doesn't
require performance. And sometimes, that community
looks different in different seasons of life, and that's okay.

What Healthy Support Can Look Like

In friendships and family, healthy support might look like people who respect your boundaries, even when they don't fully understand them. These are loved ones who don't guilt or shame you into emotional availability. People who are willing to *listen* instead of immediately trying to fix.

In hard seasons, this valuable support may look like needing space from people who trigger your old wounds. The right support system will honor your need for protection. This will require you being honest about needing more rest, more quiet, or more reassurance. Remember, it is okay to ask for help, and you can do it without apology.

And sometimes, the support you need is **professional**. A therapist who helps you process deeply rooted patterns. A coach or counselor who holds space while you build new emotional habits. A safe container where *you* don't have to be the strong one for once.

This isn't weakness or failure—it's wisdom. The kind you earn, not fake. Recognizing your need for support is not a setback. It's spiritual maturity. It's emotional intelligence. It's how we stay unbothered *without going numb*.

Final Words

You don't owe anyone your chaos. You don't have to explain your calm. You are allowed to live unbothered, deeply, fully, freely. And if you ever forget that? Come back to these pages. Come back to your breath. Come back to yourself.

You are not alone. I'm proud of you. And you've got this. **This isn't the end. It's the beginning of your unbothered era.**

ABOUT THE AUTHOR

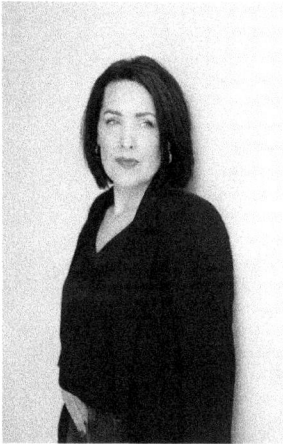

Dr. Shiloh Werkmeister helps people stop being emotionally hijacked by others so they can finally protect their peace and live with purpose.

She is a licensed psychotherapist, bestselling author, and boundary strategist who has spent over two decades helping women walk away from people-pleasing, self-doubt, and toxic cycles—and into the clarity and confidence they were made for.

After surviving abuse, burnout, and brain surgeries, Dr. Shiloh knows firsthand what it takes to rebuild your life from rock bottom. She turned her pain into purpose and created the *Unbothered* framework to help others do the same.

Today, she teaches clients, audiences, and communities how to disconnect their emotional buttons, set unapologetic boundaries, and reclaim control over their thoughts, time, and energy.

Her mission is clear: to equip cycle-breakers, empaths, and exhausted achievers with the psychological tools, spiritual grounding, and no-fluff wisdom they need to finally live free.

TAKE YOUR HEALING DEEPER

BECOMING UNBOTHERED

Join the Becoming Unbothered Program — Exclusive Offer for Readers

If this book struck a nerve (in the best way), you're not alone. You've just done the internal work of awareness, now it's time to anchor it in real life — with guidance, community, and accountability.

Becoming Unbothered is a six-week transformational journey where we walk through boundaries, emotional regulation, and detachment tools together — in real-time. It's where the book comes alive.

- Weekly coaching + curriculum

- Practical strategies and scripts

- Real-time support and community

- **Reader Bonus:** $100 off with code

UNBOTHEREDREADER

Join the waitlist for our next cohort here: https://www.drshilohspeaks.com/becoming-unbothered-waitlist

Or scan the QR Code: